Sarah Schwitalla

NFκB signaling in different stages of intestinal carcinogenesis

Sarah Schwitalla

NFκB signaling in different stages of intestinal carcinogenesis

Südwestdeutscher Verlag für Hochschulschriften

Impressum / Imprint

Bibliografische Information der Deutschen Nationalbibliothek: Die Deutsche Nationalbibliothek verzeichnet diese Publikation in der Deutschen Nationalbibliografie; detaillierte bibliografische Daten sind im Internet über http://dnb.d-nb.de abrufbar.
Alle in diesem Buch genannten Marken und Produktnamen unterliegen warenzeichen-, marken- oder patentrechtlichem Schutz bzw. sind Warenzeichen oder eingetragene Warenzeichen der jeweiligen Inhaber. Die Wiedergabe von Marken, Produktnamen, Gebrauchsnamen, Handelsnamen, Warenbezeichnungen u.s.w. in diesem Werk berechtigt auch ohne besondere Kennzeichnung nicht zu der Annahme, dass solche Namen im Sinne der Warenzeichen- und Markenschutzgesetzgebung als frei zu betrachten wären und daher von jedermann benutzt werden dürften.

Bibliographic information published by the Deutsche Nationalbibliothek: The Deutsche Nationalbibliothek lists this publication in the Deutsche Nationalbibliografie; detailed bibliographic data are available in the Internet at http://dnb.d-nb.de.
Any brand names and product names mentioned in this book are subject to trademark, brand or patent protection and are trademarks or registered trademarks of their respective holders. The use of brand names, product names, common names, trade names, product descriptions etc. even without a particular marking in this works is in no way to be construed to mean that such names may be regarded as unrestricted in respect of trademark and brand protection legislation and could thus be used by anyone.

Coverbild / Cover image: www.ingimage.com

Verlag / Publisher:
Südwestdeutscher Verlag für Hochschulschriften
ist ein Imprint der / is a trademark of
OmniScriptum GmbH & Co. KG
Heinrich-Böcking-Str. 6-8, 66121 Saarbrücken, Deutschland / Germany
Email: info@svh-verlag.de

Herstellung: siehe letzte Seite /
Printed at: see last page
ISBN: 978-3-8381-3518-2

Zugl. / Approved by: München,TU,Diss.,2013

Copyright © 2013 OmniScriptum GmbH & Co. KG
Alle Rechte vorbehalten. / All rights reserved. Saarbrücken 2013

Table of Contents

1. Introduction 5
1.1 Epidemiology of Colorectal Carcinogenesis 5
1.2 A model for colorectal carcinogenesis (Fearon & Vogelstein model) 5
1.3 Intestinal Architecture & Intestinal Stem Cells 7
1.4 30 years of Wnt 12
1.5 Wnt signaling in cancer 14
1.6 "Cell-of-origin" theory 17
1.7 Cancer Stem Cells 18
1.8 Tumor progression 20
1.9 Tumor microenvironment „the 7th hallmark of cancer" 24
1.10 NF-κB 31
1.11 NF-κB in cancer 34
1.12 p53 37

Objective of this work 40

2. Material & Methods 42
2.1 Mice 42
   2.1.1 Mouse models 42
   2.1.2 Genotyping 46
   2.1.3 AOM administration 52
   2.1.4 Tamoxifen administration 52
   2.1.5 Bone marrow transplantation 52
   2.1.6 FITC-dextran intestinal permeability test 52
   2.1.7 Depletion of intestinal microflora 53
   2.1.8 Mini endoscopy and confocal laser scanning microscopy (clsm) 53
   2.1.9 Sacrifice of mice 54
   2.1.10 Intestinal epithelial cell isolation 54
   2.1.11 Villus isolation and propagation 55
   2.1.12 Organoid culture 55
   2.1.13 Bacterial endotoxin test 56
2.2 Human Samples 56
2.3 Histology 56
   2.3.1 Haematoxylin & Eosin (H&E) staining 56
   2.3.2 Alcian Blue staining 57
   2.3.3 Azure Eosin staining 57
   2.3.4 Alkaline Phosphatase staining 58
   2.3.5 Duolink Proximity Ligation Assay 58
   2.3.6 Fluorescence in situ hybridization (FISH) 59
   2.3.7 Immunohistochemical analysis 59
   2.3.8 Digoxigenin-labeling of in situ hybridization probes 61
   2.3.9 In situ hybridization 62
   2.3.10 TUNEL staining 64

2.3.11 Tissue hypoxia detection ... 65
2.4 RNA/DNA analysis ... 66
   2.4.1 RNA Isolation ... 66
   2.4.2 cDNA Synthesis ... 66
   2.4.3 Real-Time PCR Analysis ... 67
   2.4.4 Microarray ... 71
   2.4.5 DNA isolation ... 71
   2.4.6 Array comparative genomic hybridization ... 71
2.5 Cloning ... 72
   2.5.1 Cloning of the CreER^{T2} sequence into the ER stress indicator (ERAI) plasmid ... 72
   2.5.2 Ligation of a linker oligonucleotide into a vector construct ... 74
   2.5.3 Ligation ... 74
   2.5.4 Transformation ... 74
   2.5.5 Isolation of plasmid DNA from bacteria ... 75
2.6 Chromatin Immunoprecipitation analysis (ChIP) ... 75
   2.6.1 Sequential ChIP (Re-ChIP) ... 77
2.7 Protein analysis ... 77
   2.7.1 Preparation of Protein lysates ... 77
   2.7.2 Western Blot analysis ... 78
   2.7.3 DNA Affinity Precipitation Assay (DAPA) ... 81
   2.7.4 EMSA ([γ-^{32}P] ATP radioactively labeled oligonucleotide) ... 82
   2.7.5 EMSA (3' DY682 infrared marker labeled oligonucleotide) ... 83
   2.7.6 Kinase Assay ... 84
2.8 Cell Culture ... 85
   2.8.1 Cultivation ... 85
   2.8.2 Transfection ... 85
   2.8.3 siRNA mediated knockdown ... 85
   2.8.4 Luciferase Assay ... 86
2.9 Statistics ... 86

3. Results ... 87
3.1 The role of NF-κB during tumor initiation ... 87
   3.1.1 Massive crypt compartment expansion and hyperproliferation of intestinal epithelial cells upon constitutive β-catenin activation promoted by Tnf-α dependent NF-κB activity ... 87
   3.1.2 NF-κB triggers the initiation of adenomatous cell transformation by modulating Wnt-dependent intestinal stem cell gene expression ... 89
   3.1.3 Enhanced NF-κB activity accelerates aberrant Wnt signaling-dependent crypt stem cell hyperproliferation and induces de-differentiation in non-stem cells ... 97
   3.1.4 Ex vivo dedifferentiated epithelial villus cells form spheroids with tumor stem cell capability ... 100
   3.1.5 Recombination in differentiated enterocytes leads to de-differentiation and adenoma formation in vivo ... 106
3.2 The role of NF-κB during tumor progression ... 114

3.2.1 Loss of p53 requires additional genetic mutation of Ctnnb in order to induce tumor formation and invasion *114*
3.2.2 p53 reduces the tumor incidence in Wnt- dependent tumorigenesis by inducing apoptosis and a DNA damage program in affected cells *118*
3.2.3 Loss of Tp53 leads to a myeloid cell dominated inflammatory microenvironment associated with NF-κB activation facilitating EMT and invasion *120*
3.2.4 Loss of p53 leads to intestinal barrier defect after carcinogen exposition resulting in increased bacterial translocation and serum LPS levels activating NF-κB in IEC *127*
3.2.5 IKKβ-dependent NF-κB activation generates a myeloid derived inflammatory microenvironment driving EMT and promotes aggressive tumor invasion and metastatic spread though epithelial Stat3 activation *132*
3.2.6 Tp53$^{\Delta IEC}$ mice provide a feasible system for pre-clinical examinations *138*

4. Discussion 141
4.1 NF-κB can be activated by diverse mechanisms and in turn modulates Wnt signaling by direct crosstalk with β-catenin during tumor initiation 141
4.2 NF-κB patronizes cell type plasticity during tumor initiation and during tumor progression 144
4.3 Indirect inverse crosstalk between NF-κB and p53 function reveals differing tissue specific tumor suppressive roles of p53 during tumor initiation and tumor progression 149
4.4 Intestinal microbiata has a unique tissue specific tumor promoting role 151
4.5 The TP53^{DIEC} mouse model represents the human course of colorectal cancer and is a suitable model for pre-clinical studies 153

Summary 157

Citation Index 159

Abbreviations 181

Publications 184

Danksagung 186

1. Introduction

1.1 Epidemiology of Colorectal Carcinogenesis

Colorectal cancer (CRC) is one of the major health concerns as it is the 2nd most common cause of cancer deaths in developed countries (Jemal, Siegel et al. 2009). Worldwide there are more than 1 million new diagnosed cases of colorectal cancer each year (Tenesa and Dunlop 2009).

By etiology human CRC can be classified as (1) inherited, including hereditary non-polyposis colorectal cancer due to genetic instability, and familial adenomatous polyposis coli (FAP) due to a mutation in the adenomatous polyposis coli gene, APC (Taketo and Edelmann 2009); (2) inflammatory, including Crohn's disease (CD) and ulcerative colitis (UC) (Eaden, Abrams et al. 2001); or (3) sporadic, accounting for ~80% of CRCs but with poorly defined etiology. Risk factors are mostly conditioned by environmental influences including food-borne mutagens, intestinal microfloral commensals and pathogens and chronic inflammation.

1.2 A model for colorectal carcinogenesis (Fearon & Vogelstein model)

Several early observations in human cancers (Foulds 1954) and animal models (Nowell (1976) reported that a successive accumulation of multiple genetic modifications is necessary to convert a normal human cell into a cancer cell. During the years a huge body of work has indentified thoroughly the molecular details of these observations as has been described and illustrated more concretely on the basis of colorectal cancer (Fearon and Vogelstein 1990).

The initial step in intestinal carcinogenesis involves a constitutive activation of the Wnt-pathway after stabilization of the key transcription factor β-catenin either via activating mutations in the CTNNB gene (Morin, Sparks et al. 1997) or loss of APC (Ashton-Rickardt, Dunlop et al. 1989). Accumulation of further mutations in the small GTPase KRAS amongst others are acquired in adenomas and early carcinomas while the tumor progression stage is marked by inactivating mutations in TP53 leading to invasion and metastasis formation (Fearon and Vogelstein 1990; Wood, Parsons et al. 2007).

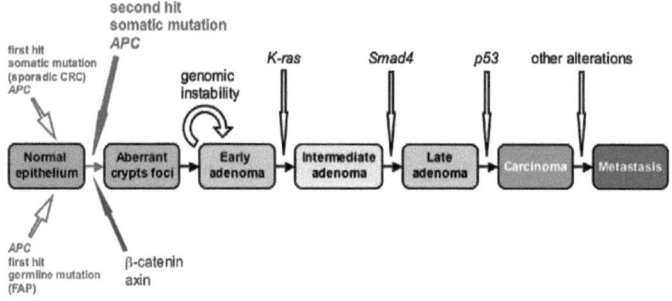

Figure 1: Accumulation of genetic changes during CRC development

Tumor initiation starts with somatic mutations in CTNNB gene or APC leading to loss of heterozygosity. Deficiency in mismatch repair enzymes (MMR) and general genomic instability speed up the tumorigenic process. Acquisition of additional mutations in indicated oncogenes and tumor suppressors is necessary to advance transformation towards a metastasising cancer cell. (Kinzler and Vogelstein 1996)

Although initiating mutations in normal epithelial or stem cells occur at low rates, mutations in APC or CTNNB are the most likely to contribute to tumor initiation. APC encodes a high molecular weight (> 300 kDa) tumor suppressor in which both alleles must be disrupted for transformation to occur. Individuals with FAP carry a mutation in one

APC allele while the 2nd allele is typically inactivated through loss of heterozygosity within the first 30 years of life, resulting in formation of multiple and aggressive tumors in the colon (Wood, Parsons et al. 2007; Taketo and Edelmann 2009). APC mutations are a prerequisite for the transition of pre-neoplastic cells to aberrant crypt foci and development of micro-adenoma towards adenoma (Korinek, Barker et al. 1997; Morin 1997). Inactivation of APC stops the differentiation and migration upwards the intestinal architecture of premalignant cells (Sansom, Reed et al. 2004), thus these cells persist in the epithelium and acquire further mutations (Network 2012) e.g. in KRAS and B-Raf, as well as in tumor suppressors, such as the TGF-b receptor (R) II (and other components of this signaling pathway), activin receptors and TP53 (Biswas, Chytil et al. 2004) for subsequent malignant conversion (Phelps, Chidester et al. 2009).

1.3 Intestinal Architecture & Intestinal Stem Cells

The epithelium of the small intestine is composed of flask-shaped submucosal invaginations known as crypts of Lieberkühn and finger-like luminal protrusions termed villi. Crypts are composed of a monoclonal, self-renewing compartment, whereas villi are characterized by differentiated cells from various lineages and are polyclonal as they receive cells from multiple crypts (Marshman, Booth et al. 2002). Crypts contain two major types of multipotent, self-renewing intestinal stem cell populations, which can be distinguished spatially by recently identified markers, the G protein-coupled receptor Lgr5 and the Polycomb group protein Bmi1 (Barker, van Es et al. 2007; Sangiorgi and Capecchi 2008). Although it is widely accepted that the intestinal stem cells that give rise to all epithelial lineages reside in the lower portions of crypts different notions in terms of numbers, exact locations and genetic signatures have been proposed. The +4 hypothesis proposes that stem cells reside at the +4 region abutting against Paneth cells (Potten, Booth et al. 1997). These cells possess unique characteristics including their high susceptibility to apoptosis, their non-random DNA strand segregation and indicated expression of marker genes such as the predominant mentioned marker Bmi1 (Sangiorgi and Capecchi 2008; Tian, Biehs et al. 2011) but also mTert (Montgomery, Carlone et al. 2011), Dclk1 (Vega, May et al. 2012) and Musashi-1 (Potten, Booth et al. 2003). In addition, the stem cell zone hypothesis argues that crypt-base columnar (CBC) cells residing at the very bottom of the crypts are the actual stem cells. Independent lineage tracing studies using Lgr5 (Barker, van Es et al. 2007), Sox9 (Furuyama, Kawaguchi et al. 2011) and Prominin-1 (Zhu, Gibson et al. 2009) have demonstrated stable labeling of the progenies of CBC cells, and a single Lgr5-high stem cell has been shown to reconstitute a long-lived and complete, self-renewing small-intestinal organoid *in vitro* (Sato, Vries et al. 2009).

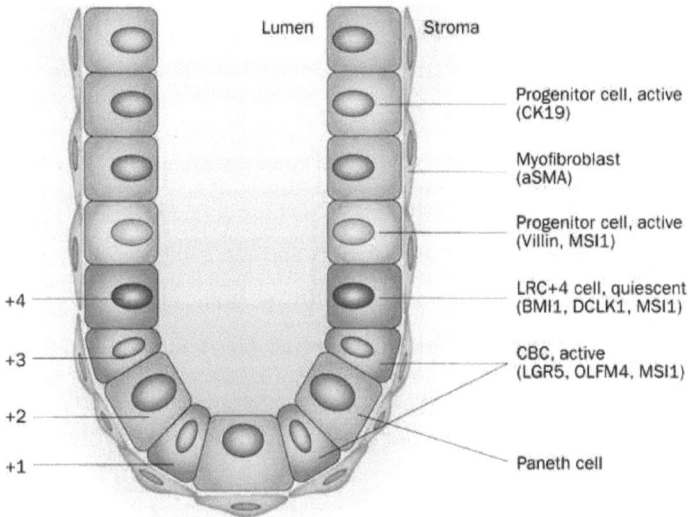

Figure 2: Location of intestinal stem cells and their markers in the intestinal crypt

Active cycling columnar crypt base cells (CBC) are intermingled with Paneth cells at the bottom of the crypt, while quiescent label retaining stem cells are located at the +4 region in the upper crypt part.
(Quante and Wang 2009)

A colored version is available in the electronic edition.

Challenging the traditional view that mammalian stem cells are slowly cycling, the discovery of Lgr5+ intestinal epithelial cells (IEC) revealed rapidly cycling crypt base columnar (CBC) cells (Barker, van Es et al. 2007) interspersed between stem cell niche feeding terminally differentiated Paneth cells (Sato, van Es et al. 2011) and are expressed throughout the intestine. Lgr5+ ISCs are equipotent and contribute to intestinal homeostasis differentiating into all intestinal cell types by neutral drift competition (Lopez-Garcia, Klein et al. 2010; Snippert, van der Flier et al. 2010; Simons and Clevers 2011). The expression of the other predominant marker Bmi1+ is mostly restricted to the "+4" crypt position abutting against the uppermost Paneth cell. Bmi1+ cells form a gradient with prevailing appearance in proximal small intestinal crypts descending towards the distal intestine (Sangiorgi and Capecchi 2008). Bmi1+ ISCs are less well characterized, however recently it has been shown that Bmi1+ ISCs represent a quiescent, injury inducible reserve ISC population being able to give rise to and repopulate LGR5+ stem cells upon damage (Yan, Chia et al. 2012). Both stem cell groups therefore mark an overlapping, interconvertible however functional different cell population indicating a bidirectional lineage relationship. The interconversion of +4 ISC and CBCs was also shown by means of another marker for quiescent +4 ISCs that express the atypical homeobox gene Hopx and give rise to Lgr5-expressing CBCs. Conversely, rapidly cycling CBCs expressing Lgr5 give rise to +4 cells expressing Hopx (Takeda, Jain et al. 2011). In a recently established single-molecule transcript counting experimental setup the installation of an expression pattern database concerning the mouse intestine demonstrated precise location of different stem cell identities. E.g. Bmi1 (Sangiorgi and Capecchi 2008), Prominin-1 (Zhu, Gibson et al. 2009) and mTert (Montgomery, Carlone et al. 2011) were expressed throughout the crypt axis at almost constant levels contrasting Lgr5 and Sox9, the expression of which was concentrated at lower crypt positions. During homeostasis the expression patterns of stem-cell markers Lgr5, Olfm4, Cd44, Ascl2 and Musashi-1, which exhibit spatially overlapping expression patterns and high single-cell correlations, are remarkably invariant, however the expression of these genes shifts towards increased expression of Ascl2, Musashi-1 and Cd44 contrasting with the almost constant levels of Lgr5 and Bmi1, when the tissue is perturbed by irradiation again indicating potential functional differences among stem-cell markers (Itzkovitz, Blat et al. 2012).

Cycling crypt stem cells give rise to distinct populations of transient-amplifying cells, on the one hand being committed to producing absorptive enterocytes and the other hand committed to producing secretory goblet cells, Paneth cells, the enteroendocrine lineage and tuft cells, a rare quiescent epithelial lineage of unknown function (Booth, Haley et al. 2000; Marshman, Booth et al. 2002; Gerbe, Brulin et al. 2009; Gerbe, van Es et al. 2011). While Paneth cells reside in the crypt base, the members of the other lineages finalize their differentiation as they migrate out of the crypt onto adjacent villi. The migration of these differentiated cells terminates at the villus tip where the cells die by apoptosis and are shed into the intestinal lumen. One cycle of total self-renewal of the intestinal epithelium is completed within 3 to 5 days (Booth, Haley et al. 2000; Marshman, Booth et al. 2002). The establishment of intestinal tissue architecture during development, proliferation and the acquisition of particular cell fates in homeostasis is coordinated by evolutionarily conserved signaling pathways, majorly the Wnt/ β -catenin (Cheng and Leblond 1974) pathway gradient in the crypts driving a genetic stem cell proliferation program (van de Wetering, Sancho et al. 2002).

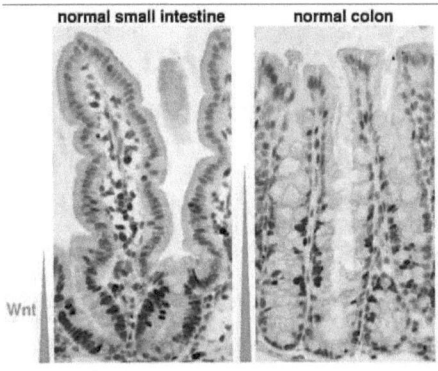

Figure 3: Cross section of small and large intestinal epithelium depicting the Wnt signaling gradient

Active Wnt signaling maintains a proliferative crypt compartment, which is responsible for the self-renewal of the whole intestinal epithelium.
(Pinto and Clevers 2005)

A colored version is available in the electronic edition.

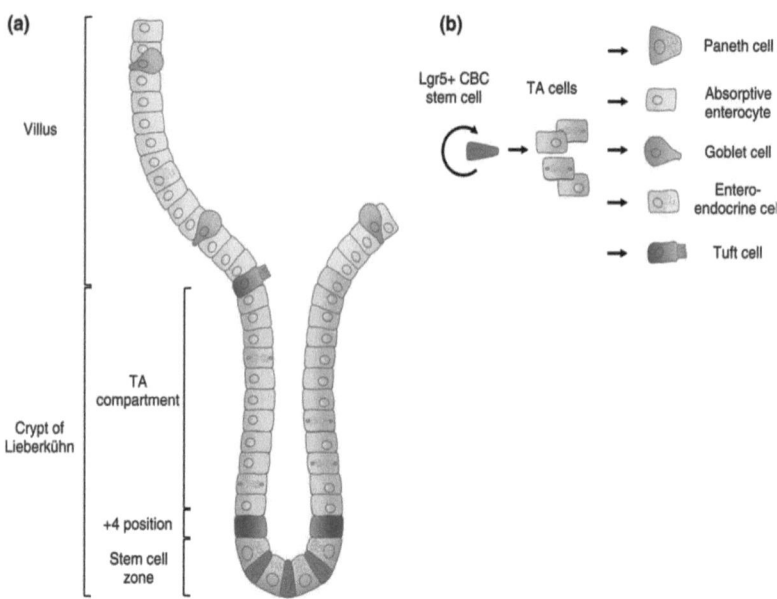

Figure 4: Model scheme of epithelial homeostasis

Cycling Lgr5+ cells (green) give rise to rapidly cycling transit amplifying cells (TA) which differentiate into enterocytes, goblet cells, enteroendocrine cells and tuft cells after passing the crypt-villus axis and migrate up to the villus tip, which they reach after 3-5days before they become shed off into the intestinal lumen. Paneth cells migrate down to the crypt base where they reside for 6-8 weeks
(Rizk and Barker 2012)

1.4 30 years of Wnt

The 'birthday' of Wnt research can be dated to 1982 when Roel Nusse and Harold Varmus reported on 'a putative proto-oncogene, transcriptionally activated by MMTV proviruses in tumors' (Nusse and Varmus 1982). Molecular cloning of the proto-oncogenic int1 locus revealed the intriguing similarity to Drosophila Wingless, a segment polarity gene discovered by developmental biologists. This convergence laid the foundation for close interactions between developmental geneticists and cancer biologists. The discovery of the first mammalian Wnt gene provided molecular evidence that cancer can arise from developmental abnormalities.

The importance of the Wnt pathway in development and tissue maintenance becomes clear from several studies e.g. inactivation of β - catenin leads to a rapid loss of intestinal epithelial cells, starting with the loss of crypts that concurs with blocked proliferation and increased enterocytic differentiation. Importantly, intestinal stem cells are induced to terminally differentiate in the absence of Wnt signaling, resulting in fatal loss of intestinal function. (Fevr, Robine et al. 2007). Blocking Wnt signaling by deletion of the TCF7L2 locus (TCF-4) depletes stem cell compartments in the intestines of mouse embryos because cells are unable to proliferate and repopulate crypts (Korinek, Barker et al. 1998).

Cytoplasmic β-catenin is the key signal transcription factor of the canonical Wnt pathway. If not bound membranously to its binding partner E-cadherin in adherens junctions in the absence of pathway stimulation by Wnt ligands, β-catenin is phosphorylated in the cytoplasm by the activity of a multiprotein destruction complex, marking β-catenin for degradation. This complex consists of the scaffold proteins Axin and Adenoma Polyposis Coli (APC), of the kinases phosphorylating β-catenin, glycogen synthase kinase 3β (GSK3β), casein kinase 1 (CK1) and protein phosphatase 2A (PP2A) (Kimelman and Xu 2006).

Upon Wnt ligand binding to Frizzled and its co-receptors LRP5/6 transmembrane receptors, the cytoplasmic protein Disheveled is recruited to the membrane complex and multimerizes building up the LRP-associated Wnt signalosome (Bilic, Huang et al. 2007). Afterwards it recruits Axin from the cytoplasmic destruction complex thereby blocking the action of the degradation complex. Unphosphorylated, unbound β-catenin is able to translocate to the nucleus and associate with TCF/LEF transcription factors, displacing Grouchos and interacting with other co-activators such as CBP or Bcl9 thus inducing transcriptional regulation of cell type specific Wnt target genes (Najdi, Holcombe et al. 2011; Archbold, Yang et al. 2012).

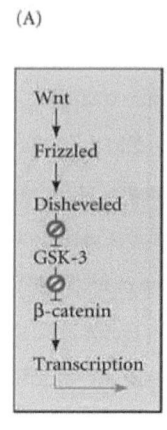
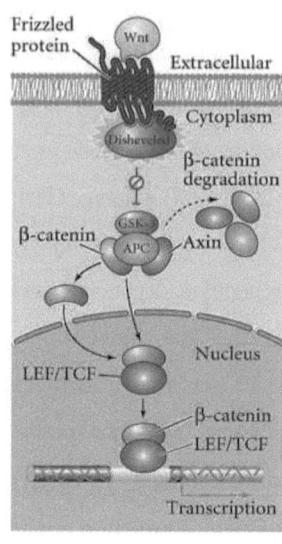

Figure 4: Wnt pathway

Upon binding of Wnt ligands to Frizzled, a receptor component assembly leads to the disruption of the cytoplasmic β-catenin destruction complex and prevents phosphorylation of β-catenin. β-catenin accumulates in the cytoplasm and translocates to the nucleus, binds to TCF/LEF cofactors and starts transcription of Wnt target genes.
(Gilbert 2010)

A colored version is available in the electronic edition

1.5 Wnt signaling in cancer

Due to its key role in regulating early cell fate decisions and adult cell homeostasis, Wnt signaling has been extensively studied for its involvement in cancer (Klaus and Birchmeier 2008).

Activation of the Wnt pathway has been related to colon cancer since the detection of truncating mutations in the tumor suppressor APC in 1989 as an early event in the carcinogenic process for sporadic and hereditary familial adenomatous polyposis (FAP) tumors (Ashton-Rickardt, Dunlop et al. 1989; Groden, Thliveris et al. 1991; Kinzler, Nilbert et al. 1991).

About 90% of sporadic colon cancers harbor activating mutations within the Wnt pathway; destroying either APC function (Miyaki, Konishi et al. 1994) or resulting in gain of function mutations of the β-catenin gene (Korinek, Barker et al. 1997; Morin, Sparks et al. 1997) preventing phosphorylation and degradation of β-catenin, leading to its accumulation. Ultimately, β-catenin translocates to the nucleus, driving persistently uncontrolled LEF/TCF-mediated gene transcription (Polakis 1999) of genes associated with the crypt stem/progenitor cell proliferation also known as the "stem cell signature" (Sansom, Reed et al. 2004; Gregorieff and Clevers 2005; Van der Flier, Sabates-Bellver et al. 2007). Intestinal crypts become enlarged as intestinal enterocytes hyperproliferate independently of their position, fail to differentiate, and no longer migrate up the crypt-villus axis (Batlle, Henderson et al. 2002; Sansom, Reed et al. 2004). In a mouse model of conditional APC loss (Sansom, Reed et al. 2004) villi were entirely populated by crypt-like cells that can be described as having a "crypt progenitor cell–like phenotype" (van de Wetering, Sancho et al. 2002). Wnt pathway mutated adenoma cells thus represent the transformed counterparts of the proliferative crypt progenitor.

Yet, activation of additional signaling pathways apart from Wnt is required for advancing adenomatous cells towards frank carcinoma (Fearon and Vogelstein 1990). For example, many sporadic colon cancers contain activating mutations in the proto-oncogenic GTPase K-RAS (40%) (Bos, Fearon et al. 1987; Forrester, Almoguera et al. 1987). Epidermal growth factor (EGF) and Vascular endothelial growth factor (VEGF) signaling can also activate Rac/K-Ras pathways, which enhance canonical Wnt signaling by increasing the residence time and concentration of β -catenin in the nucleus (Wu, Tu et al. 2008; Phelps,

Chidester et al. 2009), indicating a strong synergy between K-Ras-dependent signals and oncogenic Wnt signals. Studies on nonsteroidal anti-inflammatory drugs (NSAIDS) showing to decrease cancer risk have established a decisive role for chronic inflammation and prostaglandin signaling in colorectal tumorigenesis (Oshima and Taketo 2002; Chan, Ogino et al. 2007; Grivennikov, Greten et al. 2010) NSAIDS inhibit cyclooxygenase 2 (COX2) , which catalyzes the production of prostaglandin E 2 (PGE2). Importantly, its pharmacological inhibition negatively impacts tumor burden in colorectal cancer development (Rothwell, Fowkes et al. 2011; Chan, Arber et al. 2012). Mechanistic proposals for the interaction between prostaglandin and Wnt signaling include COX2 as a direct target gene of nuclear factor κ B (NF-κB) as well as Wnt and K-Ras signaling cooperation (Pahl 1999; Araki, Okamura et al. 2003).

Furthermore, the complex cross regulation between β -catenin signaling and the inflammation related transcription factor NF-κB is under intense investigation. Most of the models provide evidence for mechanisms of cross-regulation between Wnt and NF-κB pathways either through direct physical β-catenin and NF-κB interaction or indirectly through target gene regulation. E.g. active β-catenin signaling can elevate the expression of the β-transducing repeat containing protein (β-TrCP) mRNA and protein in a Tcf-dependent manner. β-TrCP is an E3 ubiquitin ligase receptor and targets β-catenin and inhibitor of NF-κB a (IκBα) for proteasomal degradation by specifically recognizing a 19-amino-acid destruction motif in IκB and β-catenin (Winston, Strack et al. 1999). Induction of β-TrCP expression by the β-catenin/Tcf pathway up-regulates NF-κB activity and accelerates degradation of the wild-type β-catenin, suggesting that a negative feedback loop may control the β-catenin/Tcf regulation (Spiegelman, Slaga et al. 2000).

1.6 "Cell-of-origin" theory

Although Wnt pathway activating mutations are well known for a long time to cause intestinal adenoma growth, the cell-of-origin of intestinal carcinogenesis has not been identified until 2009 (Barker, Ridgway et al. 2009). Barker et al. claim Lgr5-expressing crypt stem cells to be the tumor initiating cells. By using Lgr5 knock-in allele to delete the APC tumor suppressor in stem cells they observed rapid transformation and adenoma formation throughout the small intestine and colon (Barker, Ridgway et al. 2009). This experiment gives proof for the "Bottom-up" model of colorectal carcinogenesis claiming that transformation is initiated in a stem cell at the base of the crypt, which proliferates, replacing the normal mucosa with transformed cells from the bottom up (Preston, Wong et al. 2003). The distribution of Lgr5+ cells within stem-cell-derived adenomas indicated maintenance of stem cell/progenitor cell hierarchy in neoplastic lesions as has been predicted according to the hierarchical intestinal tissue architecture. Apart from Lgr5+ cells Bmi1+ cells are also shown to be susceptible to tumorigenesis by deregulated WNT signaling as shown in experiments using a BMI1–CreER knock-in model (Sangiorgi and Capecchi 2008; Sangiorgi and Capecchi 2009). Although the "Bottom Up" theory is the prevailing concept so far, an alternative model opposing the hierarchical unidirectional development of tumors from stem cells is arising and has been proposed formerly (Shih, Wang et al. 2001). In this so-called "Top-down" model, transformation is initiated in a differentiated cell, which spreads laterally and initiates tumor growth from the top down. Emerging evidence from multiple laboratories is beginning to support the idea that non-stem cells can dedifferentiate to form functional stem cells or Cancer Stem Cells (CSCs) as has been observed so far *in vivo* in progenitor cells reacquiring stem cell activity in mouse differentiating spermatogonia (Barroca, Lassalle et al. 2009) and in mammary luminal cells (Guo, Keckesova et al. 2012) converting to mammary stem cells by overexpressing SOX9 cooperating with Slug inducing epithelial-mesenchymal transition (EMT). Furthermore cell plasticity and bidirectional interchangeability between cancer stem cells and relatively differentiated cancer progenitors either spontaneously or under specific culture conditions has been demonstrated in several studies using immortalized or cancer cell lines (Iliopoulos, Hirsch et al. 2011) (Chaffer, Brueckmann et al. 2011; Scheel, Eaton et al. 2011).

1.7 Cancer Stem Cells

Traditionally a tumor has been considered to be a homogenous cell mass until it became more and more obvious that tumors are composed of a number of distinct clonal subpopulations. Histopathologically tumors reveal diverse regions of various degrees of differentiation, proliferation, vascularity, inflammation, and invasiveness. In recent years evidence has accumulated indicating the existence of a new dimension of intra-tumoral heterogeneity, another subclass of neoplastic cells within a tumor, termed cancer stem cells (CSCs). Traditional models of tumorigenesis suggest that every cell within the tumor population is capable of tumor initiation and propagation. The newly discussed cancer stem cells (CSC), however, propose that only a small fraction of cells possesses tumor propagation abilities (Huang and Wicha 2008). CSCs are defined through the expression of a specific set of markers that are also expressed by normal stem cells in the tissue of origin (Al-Hajj, Wicha et al. 2003) and by their ability to efficiently initiate new tumors upon inoculation into recipient host mice (Lobo, Shimono et al. 2007; Cho and Clarke 2008). Initially CSCs were implicated in the pathogenesis of hematopoietic malignancies (Bonnet and Dick 1997; Reya, Morrison et al. 2001) and were identified in solid tumors a few years later, in particular breast carcinomas and neuroectodermal tumors (Al-Hajj, Wicha et al. 2003; Gilbertson and Rich 2007). The origins of CSCs within a solid tumor have not been clarified in detail and indeed may well vary from one tumor type to another. In some tumors, normal tissue stem cells serve as the cells-of-origin that undergo oncogenic transformation to yield CSCs; in others, partially differentiated transit-amplifying cells or even differentiated cells may suffer the initial oncogenic transformation by obtaining more stem-like character.

Three recent independent lineage tracing studies of mouse models of brain (Chen, Li et al. 2012), skin (Driessens, Beck et al. 2012) and intestinal (Schepers, Snippert et al. 2012) tumors provide the first evidence that CSCs do exist and arise de novo during tumor formation in intact organs. Of note, by "lineage retracing" using the multicolor Cre-reporter R26R-Confetti, Schepers et al. demonstrate that the crypt stem cell marker Lgr5 also marks a subpopulation of adenoma cells that fuel the growth of established intestinal adenomas. These Lgr5+ cells, which represent about 5 to 10% of the cells in the adenomas, generate additional Lgr5+ cells as well as all other adenoma cell types (Schepers, Snippert et al. 2012). Considering that adenomas are still similarly organized as the corresponding normal tissue, it is expected that these benign tumors contain cell hierarchies that approximate to normality. However, there is evidence for a hierarchical structure in malignant tumors as well, as Chen et al. are able to demonstrate that CSCs repopulate the tumor after it has been eradicated by anti-cancer drugs, whereas tumor burden could be dramatically decreased by targeting CSC additionally (Chen, Li et al. 2012).

Moreover recent studies related the acquisition of CSC traits with the EMT trans-differentiation program during tumor progression (Mani, Guo et al. 2008; Morel, Lievre et al. 2008; Singh and Settleman 2010). This analogy suggests that the EMT may enable cancer cells to physically disseminate from primary tumors but additionally it can confer the self-renewal capability and subsequent clonal expansion at sites of dissemination on such cells (Brabletz, Jung et al. 2005). Signals released by an activated, inflammatory stroma that trigger an EMT, may also be important in creating and maintaining CSC.

1.8 Tumor progression

According to the genetic model of colorectal carcinogenesis proposed in 1990 by Eric Fearon and Bert Vogelstein (Fearon and Vogelstein 1990) tumorigenesis is intiated by mutations in the Wnt pathway whereas tumor progression and the development of invasive cancer can primarily be attributed to inactivating mutations in TP53 (Fearon and Vogelstein 1990; Wood, Parsons et al. 2007). The molecular mechanisms underlying invasion and metastasis still remain a subject of study. It can be observed that as carcinomas arising from epithelial tissues and progressing to more malignant pathological grades the affected cancer cells typically develop alterations in their morphology as well as in their attachment to other cells and to the extracellular matrix (ECM). The best-characterized alteration involved the loss of E-cadherin, a key cell-to cell adhesion molecule. By forming adherens junctions with adjacent epithelial cells, E-cadherin helps to assemble epithelial cell sheets and maintainance of the cells within these sheets. Increased expression of E-cadherin antagonizes invasion and metastasis, whereas reduction of its expression is known to potentiate these abilities. The frequently observed downregulation and occasional mutational inactivation of E-cadherin in human carcinomas provided strong support for its role as a key suppressor of epithelial-mesenchymal transition (EMT) (Cavallaro and Christofori 2004; Berx and van Roy 2009). The multistep process of invasion and metastasis is accomplished by a complex succession of cell biological events — collectively termed the invasion-metastasis cascade - whereby epithelial cells in primary tumors invade locally through surrounding extracellular matrix (ECM) and stromal cell layers, intravasate into the lumina of blood vessels, survive the transport through the vasculature, arrest at distant organ sites, extravasate into the parenchyma of distant tissues, initially survive in these foreign microenvironments in order to form micrometastases, and reinitiate their proliferative programs at metastatic sites, thereby generating macroscopic clinically detectable metastatic colonies (Fidler and Kripke 2003).

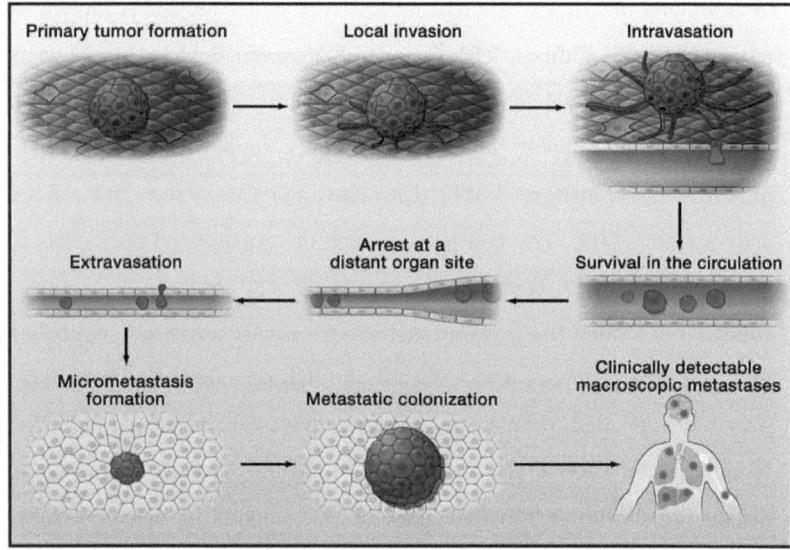

Figure 5: The Invasion-Metastasis cascade

After tumor invasion tumor cell colonies intravasate and start circulation to distant organ sites. A prerequisite for systemic translocation is their survival in the circulation and arrest at the target organ. The tumor cell colonies extravasate into the tissue and take advantage of the local microenvironment to persist and induce metastatic growth. (Valastyan and Weinberg 2011)

A colored version is available in the electronic edition

Many of these complex cellular events are orchestrated by molecular pathways within carcinoma cells. Importantly, carcinoma cells additionally enlist non-neoplastic stromal cells to aid in and support each step of the invasion-metastasis cascade in a cell non-autonomous manner.

''Epithelial-mesenchymal transition'' (EMT), known as a developmental regulatory program, has become prominently implicated as a mechanism by which transformed epithelial cells can acquire the abilities to invade, to resist apoptosis, and to disseminate (Barrallo-Gimeno and Nieto 2005; Klymkowsky and Savagner 2009; Polyak and Weinberg 2009; Thiery, Acloque et al. 2009; Yilmaz and Christofori 2009). This multifaceted

EMT program can be activated transiently or stably by carcinoma cells in various extent during the course of invasion and metastasis. A set of pleiotropically acting transcriptional factors, including Snail, Slug, Twist, and Zeb1/2 was initially identified in developmental genetics to control EMT and related migratory processes during embryogenesis. These EMT regulators are expressed in a number of malignant tumor types as well and have been shown in mouse models of carcinoma formation to be causally important for programming invasion; some have been found to elicit metastasis when ectopically overexpressed (Yang and Weinberg 2008; Schmalhofer, Brabletz et al. 2009; Micalizzi, Farabaugh et al. 2010). Included in EMT regulating transcription factor overexpression is loss of adherens junctions and associated conversion from an epithelial to a spindle shaped, fibroblastic morphology, expression of matrix-degrading enzymes, increased motility, and heightened resistance to apoptosis. Snail can directly repress the E-cadherin gene expression, thereby depriving neoplastic epithelial cells of this key suppressor of motility and invasiveness (Peinado, Ballestar et al. 2004). So far no evidence has been given to describe the EMT transcription factor interactions and the conditions that govern their expression. Developmental genetics indicate that contextual signals received from neighboring cells in the embryo are involved in triggering expression of these transcription factors in those cells destined to pass through an EMT (Micalizzi, Farabaugh et al. 2010); analogously, increasing evidence suggests that interactions of cancer cells with adjacent tumor-associated stromal cells can induce expression of the malignant cell phenotypes that are known to be choreographed by EMT controlling factors (Brabletz, Jung et al. 2001; Karnoub, Dash et al. 2007). Moreover, cancer cells at the invasive front can be seen to have undergone an EMT, suggesting that these cancer cells are subject to microenvironmental stimuli distinct from those received by cancer cells located in the cores of these lesions (Hlubek, Brabletz et al. 2007). Although the evidence is still incomplete, it appears that EMT-inducing transcription factors are able to orchestrate most steps of the invasion-metastasis cascade. Additionally, it remains to be determined whether invasive carcinoma cells necessarily acquire their capability through activation of the EMT program, or whether alternative regulatory programs can also enable this capability. For sure, crosstalk between cancer cells and cells of the neoplastic stroma is involved in the acquired capability for invasive growth and metastasis (Kalluri and Zeisberg 2006; Joyce and Pollard 2009; Egeblad, Nakasone et al. 2010; Qian and Pollard 2010). Tumor associated macrophages at the tumor periphery can support local invasion by supplying matrix-degrading enzymes such as metalloproteinases and cysteine cathepsin proteases (Mohamed and Sloane 2006; Palermo and Joyce 2008; Joyce and Pollard 2009; Kessenbrock, Plaks et al. 2010). These observations indicate that the malignant phenotypes do not arise in a strictly cell-autonomous manner.

1.9 Tumor microenvironment „the 7th hallmark of cancer"

Since Rudolf Virchow's early finding of the presence of leukocytes within tumors in the 19th century, the important link between inflammation and tumor development has already been suggested and is a well accepted fact today. While only the minority of tumors is caused by germline mutations, the majority of tumors is caused by somatic mutations and environmental factors (90%) such as chronic inflammatory conditions. In several types of inflammatory diseases such as chronic hepatitis or inflammatory bowel disease (IBD) chronic inflammatory conditions have been shown to increase cancer risk and act pro-tumorigenic (Pikarsky, Porat et al. 2004; Waldner and Neurath 2009; Grivennikov, Greten et al. 2010).

Inflammation and its establishment of a tumor microenvironment can be evident at the earliest stages of neoplastic progression and is demonstrably capable of fostering the development of incipient neosplasia into full-blown cancers. Due to relative similarity to wound-healing situations with continuous cell proliferation induced by an inflammatory microenvironment tumors were regarded as "wounds that do not heal" since the 1980s (Dvorak 1986). Due to its multiple influential contributions to all important steps in carcinogenesis, tumor microenvironment has recently been accepted as a hallmark into the model principle of "the hallmarks of cancer" providing a framework for understanding the progression of a normal cell towards a neoplastic state by acquiring a number of hallmark capabilities besides the stepwise accumulation of activating mutations (Hanahan and Weinberg 2000; Hanahan and Weinberg 2011).

Tumor initiation may be enhanced by the production of growth factors and cytokines promoting proliferation of tumor progenitors or stimulation of stem cell expansion. Indeed, NF-κB enhances Wnt/β-catenin signaling in colonic crypts (Umar, Sarkar et al. 2009). The pro-inflammatory NF-κB target TNF-α can promote nuclear shuttling of β-catenin during inflammation-associated gastric cancer even in the absence of Wnt/β-catenin pathway mutations (Oguma, Oshima et al. 2008). Yet, the role of inflammation on early tumor initiation has not been addressed molecularly. The first genetic evidence for inflammatory cells as a source of tumor-promoting cytokines was shown in a mouse model of colitis associated carcinogenesis (CAC), where inactivation of NF-κB in myeloid cells reduced tumor growth and blocked production of IL-6 and other cytokines in response to colitis whereas NF-κB in epithelial cells promoted cell survival of affected cells (Greten, Eckmann et al. 2004). The influence of immune cells in CAC was furthermore shown to be mediated through other pro-inflammatory microenvironmental markers such as IL-6, IL-11, TNF-α, and IL-1β, as well as IL-23 (Becker, Fantini et al. 2004; Popivanova, Kitamura et al. 2008; Bollrath, Phesse et al. 2009; Grivennikov, Karin et al. 2009; Kortylewski, Xin et al. 2009).

The microenvironment acts as a communicational platform for diverse cells among each other by means of mostly cytokine and chemokine production and act in autocrine and paracrine manners to control and educate tumors. Infiltrating cells fostering the tumor microenvironment comprise the innate immune system including macrophage subtypes, neutrophils, mast cells, myeloid-derived suppressor cells, dendritic cells as well as natural killer cells and adaptive immune cells including T and B lymphocytes in addition to the cancer cells and their surrounding stroma consisting of fibroblasts, endothelial cells, pericytes, and mesenchymal cells (de Visser, Eichten et al. 2006).

Considering the contrary functions of the immune system, on the one hand detecting and targeting infectious agents with the adaptive immune response, which is supported by cells of the innate immune system and on the other hand involvement in wound healing and clearing of dead cells and cellular debris, one can relate the counterintuitive existence of both tumor-promoting and tumor-antagonizing immune cells. Molecules and microenvironmental conditions, such as a specific cytokine pattern and hypoxia, present within the tumor microenvironment have the capacity to pilot recruitment, maturation and differentiation of infiltrating leukocytes and play a central role in their functional plasticity away from anti-tumor functions promoting their pro-tumoral function (Pollard 2004). Tumor modulating functions are accomplished by distinct subclasses of inflammatory cells, namely a class of conventional macrophages (M1) and neutrophils supporting adaptive immunity of B and T cells, and subclasses of alternatively activated macrophages (M2), neutrophils, and myeloid progenitors that are engaged in wound healing and neoplastic progression (Johansson, Denardo et al. 2008; Egeblad, Nakasone et al. 2010; Mantovani 2010; Qian and Pollard 2010).

Whereas the polarization of neutrophils still remains to be elusive, macrophage polarization and analogously T-cell polarization have been studied in detail and regarded as among the most important players in cancers (Solinas, Germano et al. 2009) Pro-tumoral tumor associated macrophages (TAMs) have decreased ability to present tumor-associated antigens, lyse tumor cells, and stimulate the anti-tumor functions of T-cells and NK cells (Mantovani, Sozzani et al. 2002). Unlike Th1 and Th2 cells, M1 and M2 macrophages are plastic and their phenotype is defined by their gene expression prolife rather than by deterministic differentiation pathways and lineage choices. TAMs are composed of several distinct populations that often share features of classically activated pro- inflammatory M1 macrophages and an alternatively activated pro- tumorigenic M2 macrophage phenotype (Mantovani, Sozzani et al. 2002), but with greater overall similarity to macrophages involved in developmental processes (Ojalvo, King et al. 2009; Ojalvo, Whittaker et al. 2010). All of these macrophage subtypes are defined by the expression of the canonical markers CD11b, F4/80, and colony stimulating factor 1 receptor (CSF-1R), as well as absence of Gr1 (Ly6G), but they are educated by microenvironmental cues to adopt a particular phenotype expressing different cytokine patterns either regulating inflammation, immune regulation, angiogenesis, invasion, intravasation or metastasis (Qian and Pollard 2010). In specific, M1 macrophages are activated by IFNg and microbial products and express high levels of pro-inflammatory cytokines (TNF-α, IL-1, IL-6, IL-12 or IL-23), major histocompatibility complex (MHC) molecules, and inducible nitric oxide synthase. By contrast, M2 or "alternatively" activated Macrophages are induced by IL-4, IL-10, and IL-13, downregulate MHC class II and IL-12 and show increased expression of the anti-inflammatory cytokine IL-10, scavenger receptor A, and arginase. Over-expression of IL-10, TGF-b and prostaglandins is believed to contribute to the immunosuppressive phenotype via activating immune- suppressive T regulatory cells (T_{regs}) and blocking of T-cell mediated anti-tumor activity which is associated with increased tumor growth (Sica, Saccani et al. 2000; Mantovani, Sozzani et al. 2002; Sakaguchi 2005; Smyth, Teng et al. 2006). In addition it was shown that HIF-1a activated in TAMs by hypoxia influences the positioning and function of tumor cells, stromal cells, and TAMs by selectively upregulating the expression of CXC chemokine receptor 4 (CXCR4) and CXCR4 ligand which is involved in cancer metastases conferring TAMs a major role in advanced tumor stages (Muller, Homey et al. 2001; Schioppa, Uranchimeg et al. 2003; Ceradini, Kulkarni et al. 2004). It has been reported that over 80% of studies show a correlation between macrophage density and poor patient prognosis (Bingle, Brown et al. 2002).

In the same way T cells can exhibit both tumor-suppressive and -promoting effects, as determined by their effector functions (DeNardo, Andreu et al. 2010) (Smyth, Dunn et al. 2006; Langowski, Kastelein et al. 2007). Mature T cells can be classified into two major groups according to their respective T cell receptors (TCRs) gd and ab. ab-T cells can be subdivided as CD8+ cytotoxic T cells (CTLs) and CD4+ helper T (Th) cells including Th1, Th2, Th17, and T regulatory (T_{reg}) cells, as well as natural killer T (NKT) cells. Similar to TAMs, the tumor-promoting and anti-tumorigenic functions of T lymphocytes are mediated by cytokines and cytotoxic mechanisms (Lin and Karin 2007; Swann and Smyth 2007). Increased numbers of activated CTLs including CD8+ T cells and IFNg-producing Th1 cells, correlate with better survival in some cancers, including invasive colon cancer, melanoma, multiple myeloma, and pancreatic cancer (Galon, Costes et al. 2006; Swann and Smyth 2007; Laghi, Bianchi et al. 2009). Importantly, the adaptive transfer of CD4+ CD25+ Regulatory T cells to Apc^{Min} mice dramatically reduced the number of intestinal polyps, with the induction of tumor cell necrosis (Erdman, Sohn et al. 2005; Gounaris, Blatner et al. 2009), which was not the case when cells are prepared from IL10-/- mice (Erdman, Rao et al. 2003). However, many of the T cell subsets found in solid tumors, act pro-tumorigenic supporting tumor promotion, progression, or metastasis including Th2 cells (Aspord, Pedroza-Gonzalez et al. 2007; DeNardo, Barreto et al. 2009), and Th17 cells (Langowski, Zhang et al. 2006). In breast cancer, a high CD4+/CD8+ and Th2/Th1 ratio of infiltrated T cells is indicative of poor prognosis (Kohrt, Nouri et al. 2005). Th2 CD4+T cells are able to educate TAMs to produce proangiogenic and prometastatic factors (DeNardo, Barreto et al. 2009). In colitis-associated cancer (CAC), infiltrating T cells also appear to play a tumor-promoting function (Waldner and Neurath 2009).

In addition to fully differentiated immune cells present in tumor stroma, a variety of partially differentiated myeloid progenitors have been identified in tumors (Murdoch, Muthana et al. 2008). Myeloid progenitors represent intermediaries between circulating bone marrow originated cells and the differentiated immune cells usually found in normal and inflamed tissues. Importantly, these progenitors have considerable tumor-promoting activity like their differentiated counterparts. Of particular interest, a class of tumor infiltrating myeloid cells co-expressing the macrophage marker CD11b and the neutrophil marker Gr1 has been shown to suppress anti-tumorigenic CD8+ cytotoxic T lymphocytes and natural killer (NK) cell activity. Independently these cells have been identified as actively immune-suppressive myeloid-derived suppressor cells (MDSCs) along with regulatory T cells (Tregs) suppressing the action of cytotoxic lymphocytes (Ostrand-Rosenberg and Sinha 2009; Mougiakakos, Choudhury et al. 2010; Qian and Pollard 2010).

The inflammatory microenvironment is fuelled by growth factors such as EGF that sustain proliferative signaling to the tumor microenvironment, release of chemicals, notably reactive oxygen species, that have further mutagenic and tumor promoting effect for nearby cells, secretion of survival factors that limit cell death. Different cytokines can either promote or inhibit tumor development and progression (Lin and Karin 2007). Through activation of various key signaling components including NF-κB, AP-1, STAT, and SMAD transcription factors, as well as caspases, cytokines are responsible to control either antitumor immunity (IL-12, TRAIL, IFNg) or enhance tumor progression (IL-6, IL-17, IL-23) by favoring tumor cell growth and survival (TRAIL, FasL, TNF-α, EGFR ligands, TGF-b, IL-6). For instance, IL-10, expressed by regulatory T cells, suppresses intestinal tumorigenesis by inhibiting the formation of the inflammatory network during tumor initiation in APC^{min} mice (Erdman, Poutahidis et al. 2003; Erdman, Rao et al. 2003), conversely it was observed that CD25+ Foxp3+ T$_{reg}$ cells performed a switch from IL-10 expression to the production of pro-inflammatory IL-17 in polyp tissue supporting tumor development (Colombo and Piconese 2009). Advanced tumor growth requires the induction of tumor vasculature, termed the "angiogenic switch" triggered by hypoxia (Bergers and Benjamin 2003). Tumor hypoxia promotes angiogenesis and increases the probability of metastasis. Tumor angiogenesis depends on recruitment of tumor- associated macrophages (TAMs) by angiopoetin 2 and vascular endothelial growth factor (VEGF), which sense hypoxic signals and in turn produce chemokines and proangiogenic factors. Importantly, expression of pro-angiogenic genes, such as IL-8, CXCL1, CXCL8, VEGF, FGF2, hypoxia-inducible factor 1 alpha (HIF-1a), and pro-invasive extracellular matrix-degrading enzymes like matrix metalloproteinases (MMPs) as well as cathepsin proteases facilitate activation of epithelial- mesenchymal- transition (EMT), invasion, and metastasis (Karnoub, Dash et al. 2007; DeNardo, Andreu et al. 2010; Grivennikov, Greten et al. 2010; Qian and Pollard 2010) are directly regulated by NF-κB, STAT3, and AP-1 in TAMs, MDSCs, and other cell types (Kujawski, Kortylewski et al. 2008; Rius, Guma et al. 2008).

1.10 NF-κB

Since the major transcription factor involved in the establishment of a tumor promoting microenvironment during the carcinogenic process is NF-κB, it can be regarded as a non-classical oncogene, whose activation in malignant cells is predominantly dependent on external signals produced by neighboring cells. NF-κB controls cell survival, proliferation, and growth, as well as angiogenesis, invasiveness, motility, chemokine, and cytokine production (Yu, Pardoll et al. 2009; Grivennikov and Karin 2010).

NF-κB is one of the best-studied transcription factors. This is evident from the fact that although NF-κB was discovered only 25 years ago (Sen and Baltimore 1986) and makes up one of ~2000 estimated transcription factors in humans (Lander, Linton et al. 2001; GuhaThakurta 2006), ~10% of research articles listed in PubMed on the subject of transcription factors are associated with NF-κB. Around half of the published articles highlight its importance in tumor development. As NF-κB is the key transcription factor involved in the inflammatory pathway, it is constitutively active in most cancers and many of the signaling pathways implicated in cancer are connected to the activation of NF-κB (Grivennikov, Greten et al. 2010; Grivennikov and Karin 2010). Mammalian NF-κB is a family of transcription factors including five members: RelA/p65, c-Rel, RelB, NF-κB1 (p50) and NF-κB2 (p52) (Ghosh and Karin 2002; Vallabhapurapu and Karin 2009). NF-κB dimer complexes are associated with their inhibitors, IκB proteins. There are diverse human IκB proteins, including IκBα, IκBβ, IκBε and IκBζ. In addition, the precursor full-length proteins p105 and p100 as well as their processed forms p50 and p52 also function as IκB proteins. The principal inactive form of the NF-κB complex is a p50–p65 (RelA)–IκBa trimer, located in the cytoplasm. In the classic or canonical pathway, in response to various external stimuli, IκBa is phosphorylated at Ser 32 and Ser 36 by the IκBα kinase (IKK) complex, which is a complex of three proteins, two catalytic (IKKα and IKKβ) and one regulatory (IKKγ, also known as the NF-κB essential modulator (NEMO)). The IKK complex finally modifies IKKγ by phosphorylation and K-63 ubiquitinylation (Perkins 2006; Scheidereit 2006; Bhoj and Chen 2009; Chen and Sun 2009). Phosphorylation of IkBa promotes K-48 ubiquitination of IκBa by the SCF– bTrCP complex and its degradation by the proteasome. The released NF-κB dimer p50–p65 is also phosphorylated by IKK and furthermore is translocated to the nucleus, where it binds to response elements in its promoters to activate the transcription of responsive genes (Vallabhapurapu and Karin 2009). At the NF-κB responsive promoters, the p65 subunit of NF-κB is further modified by acetylation and methylation, and it interacts with additional coactivators (Werner, Barken et al. 2005).

The non-canonical or alternative pathway involves processing of p100 to p52 after phosphorylation at Ser 866 and Ser 870 by IKKα regulated by SUMOylation. IKKα is activated via NIK, which is subject to receptor-induced stabilization in the cytoplasm. The resulting NF-κB, dimer composed of processed p52 complexing RelB, migrates to the nucleus and regulates transcription of its target genes (Senftleben, Cao et al. 2001; Vatsyayan, Qing et al. 2008).

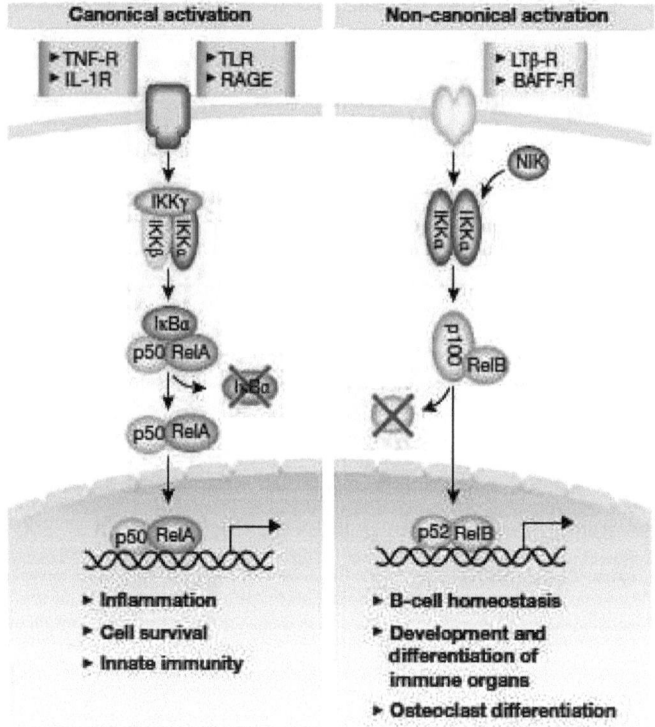

Figure 6: NF-κB pathway

In response to different stimuli canonical, dependent on IKKβ and IKKγ, or non-canonical NF-κB signaling, based on IKKα activity, can be activated leading to a release of a respective NF-κB dimer which translocates to the nucleus in order to transcribe genes related to inflammation and cell survival in terms of canonical signaling, while non-classical signaling is mostly active during differentiation and immune homeostatic processes.
(Bollrath and Greten 2009)

1.11 NF-κB in cancer

Besides having a role in regulating adaptive immune response, NF-κB signaling also has a critical role in cancer development and progression (Aggarwal 2004; Basseres and Baldwin 2006; Karin 2006; Mantovani,

Allavena et al. 2008; Prasad, Ravindran et al. 2010). The production of tumor-promoting cytokines by immune/inflammatory cells that activate transcription factors such as NF-κB, STAT3 and AP1 induces genes responsible for cell proliferation, survival, angiogenesis and metastasis (Grivennikov, Greten et al. 2010). Aberrant constitutive activation of NF-κB has been observed in a variety of malignancies such as hematological, gastrointestinal, genitourinary, gynecological, thoracic, head and neck, and breast tumors and in melanoma and fibrosarcoma (Prasad, Ravindran et al. 2010). Activated NF-κB was initially described in lymphoid cancers and is detected in most solid tumors as well (Karin, Cao et al. 2002).

A number of mechanisms have been ascribed to the constitutive activation of NF-κB in cancers. Autocrine and paracrine secretion of inflammatory chemokines and cytokines such as tumor necrosis factor a (TNF-α) and IL-1b have been shown to activate NF-κB constitutively in head and neck cancer cells, acute myeloid leukemia, T-cell lymphoma and breast cancer (Giri and Aggarwal 1998; Estrov, Shishodia et al. 2003; Jackson-Bernitsas, Ichikawa et al. 2007; Braunstein, Formenti et al. 2008). Another mechanism that is implicated in the constitutive activation of NF-κB is mutations and overexpression of ligands and receptors such as epidermal growth factor (EGF) (Sethi, Ahn et al. 2007), HER-2/Neu (Pianetti, Arsura et al. 2001; Le Page, Koumakpayi et al. 2005), hepatocyte growth factors (HGF) (Fan, Gao et al. 2005) and integrins (Guo and Giancotti 2004). Several mutationally activated cell signaling pathways have been investigated to network with aberrant NF-κB. Overexpression of G-protein coupled receptors H- and K-Ras was shown to contribute to the malignant phenotype in head and neck squamous cell carcinoma (Vitale-Cross, Amornphimoltham et al. 2004; Hunter, Parkinson et al. 2005; Lu, Herrington et al. 2006; Thomas, Bhola et al. 2006; Patel, Rosenfeldt et al. 2007). In lung cancer, activating mutations of the protein kinases EGFR, ERBB2 and BRAF have been reported (Brose, Volpe et al. 2002; Naoki, Chen et al. 2002; Sanchez-Cespedes, Parrella et al. 2002; Paez, Janne et al. 2004; Stephens, Hunter et al. 2004). Furthermore several tumor suppressor genes were inactivated, including TP53 (80–90% of cases), RB1 (60–90% of cases) and PTEN (13% of cases). Epidermal growth factor and EGFR pathways (Ras–Raf–MEK) (Duffy and Kummar 2009) have been shown to activate NF-κB through Akt activation as well as through direct tyrosine phosphorylation of IkBa (Sethi, Ahn et al. 2007). The PI3K–Akt signaling pathway, induced by EGFR and Her-2, is involved in the constitutive activation of NF-κB in prostate cancer cell lines (Koumakpayi, Le Page et al. 2010). GSK3b, another kinase, is shown to regulate activation of NF-κB as genetic disruption of GSK3b abrogates TNF-α- or IL-1β-induced NF-κB activation (Hoeflich, Luo et al. 2000). In addition GSK3β activates a subset of NF-κB responsive genes by phosphorylating p65 at Ser 468 (Steinbrecher, Wilson et al. 2005). With use of lung cell lines expressing oncogenic K-Ras, NF-κB has been shown to be activated in these cells in a K-Ras-dependent manner, and this activation by K-Ras has been shown to require IKKB kinase activity. Interaction between K-Ras, TP53 and NF-κB signaling was demonstrated in mouse model of lung adenocarcinoma (Meylan, Dooley et al. 2009). Of interest, hypoxia induced activation of NF-κB in fetal lung fibroblasts also involved phosphorylation of IkBa at Tyr 42 residues (Wright, Zhuang et al. 2009). Therefore, presumably a hypoxic tumor environment may activate NF-κB as well. Activated NF-κB (p50–p65) cooperates with many other transcription factors to form on and off promoter complexes, such as STAT3 (Grivennikov and Karin 2010), SP1 (Perkins,

Edwards et al. 1993), and HIF-1α (Scortegagna, Cataisson et al. 2008).

1.12 p53

The transcription factor p53 is a key player in preventing DNA damage, for which it has earned the nickname 'guardian of the genome' (Lane 1992). The p53 network has been studied extensively over the last three decades since its discovery in 1979 (DeLeo, Jay et al. 1979). At that time retroviruses were known to promote neoplastic transformation by overexpressing 'hijacked' cancer-promoting cellular proteins. Several groups independently realized that when sera from animals with SV40 virus -induced tumors were used to immunoprecipitate SV40 large T-antigen, a non-viral protein with an apparent molecular mass of around 53 kDa was present. During the first years after its discovery, p53 was believed to be an oncogene but only in the early part of the last decade of the twentieth century, p53 has been conferred the role as a major tumor suppressor.

The level of p53 in the cell underlies a dynamic oscillating equilibrium. p53 is expressed ubiquitously as an inactive protein that has a very short half-life (20–30 min) and is present at low levels in unstressed cells. In response to strong cellular stresses, such as DNA damage or oncogenic signals, the wild-type form of p53, after it is post-translationally modified and stabilized, regulates expression of a large cohort of genes that effect reversible cell-cycle arrest in G1 or G2 phases, senescence, and apoptosis (Levine 1997; Oren 2003; Levine, Hu et al. 2006). The response to p53 activation is variable and highly dependent on both the type of cell and the nature of the damaging agent and cellular stress. This cytostatic activity of p53 can presumably contribute to tumor suppression; either by preventing the accumulation of oncogenic lesions or by eradicating damaged cells through cell death or senescence. Recent findings have uncovered additional roles of the p53 protein that is expressed under basal physiologic and cell-culture stress conditions, notably regulation of mitochondrial respiration (Bensaad, Tsuruta et al. 2006; Matoba, Kang et al. 2006), autophagy (Crighton, Wilkinson et al. 2006), and protection of the genome from reactive oxygen species (Sablina, Budanov et al. 2005). The frequencies of reported TP53 mutations vary considerably between cancer types, ranging from ~10% in haematopoietic malignancies (Peller and Rotter 2003) to 50–70% in ovarian (Schuijer and Berns 2003), colorectal (Iacopetta 2003) and head and neck (Blons and Laurent-Puig 2003). Whereas somatic TP53 mutations contribute to sporadic cancer, germline TP53 mutations cause a rare type of cancer predisposition known as Li–Fraumeni Syndrome (LFS) (Malkin, Li et al. 1990). Importantly, both somatic and germline TP53 mutations are usually followed by loss of heterozygosity (LOH) during tumor progression, which suggests that a selective force inactivates the remaining wild-type allele. The majority of TP53 mutations observed in human cancers abrogate the sequence-specific DNA-binding activity towards the wild-type p53 responsive element (Kato, Han et al. 2003), thereby lose their tumor suppressive function, acquire dominant-negative activities and gain new oncogenic properties that are independent of wild-type p53 (Wolf, Harris et al. 1984; Shaulsky, Goldfinger et al. 1991; Dittmer, Pati et al. 1993).

The variety of different responses highlights the complex role of p53 in guarding health of cells on the one hand but also in supporting tumorigenesis by a number of actions. Improperly regulated activities that normally contribute to tumor suppression might help to switch p53's role towards promotion of cancer development. This includes the pro-survival functions of p53, which might protect cells undergoing repair following stress but would be counterproductive if maintained in irreparably damaged cells. For instance, the ability of p53 to impede glycolysis can help control oncogenic transformation, but the consequent promotion of alternative metabolic pathways might also drive the anabolism necessary for tumor cell growth (DeBerardinis, Lum et al. 2008).

Objective of this work

Colorectal cancer (CRC) remains one of the world leading health problems among industrialized countries. About 608 000 deaths from colorectal cancer are estimated worldwide per year, rendering it one of the most common causes of death from cancer. A widely studied pharmacologic agent for the prevention of CRC in humans is aspirin. Data resulting from several meta- studies and epidemiologic observations provide considerable evidence that longterm administration of non-steroidal anti-inflammatory drugs (NSAID) reduces the incidence of colorectal neoplasia and is even associated with reduced CRC mortality indicating that inflammatory pathways play a crucial role already during tumor initiation but associated mechanisms remain elusive so far. NF-κB, one of the major inflammation associated transcription factors, is found to be constitutively active in most cancers. Its participation during tumor promotion leading to tumor progression has been studied in the context of chronic inflammatory conditions rather than in sporadic tumor induction, although 80% of CRC cases are attributed to a sporadic origin. According to the genetic model of colorectal carcinogenesis by Eric Fearon and Bert Vogelstein, tumorigenesis is intiated by mutations in the Wnt pathway whereas tumor progression and the development of invasive cancer can primarily be attributed to inactivating mutations in TP53. Although recent genetic studies have confirmed that TP53 is one of the most commonly mutated genes in human colorectal cancer, functional evidence due to lacking appropriate *in vivo* mouse models supporting a substantial role for p53 to specifically suppress colorectal tumor invasion is still missing.

The aim of the study is to understand the role of NF-κB during tumor initiation using a mouse model exhibiting a constitutively active Wnt pathway in intestinal epithelial cells (IEC). To examine the cell type specific functions of NF-κB and the mechanisms of sporadic colorectal tumor progression mice having an IEC specific deletion of p53 (Tp53^{DIEC}) are used as a model.

2. Material & Methods

2.1 Mice

2.1.1 Mouse models

Apc^{580S} (Shibata, Toyama et al. 1997)

Exon 14 within the APC gene is flanked by loxP sites resulting in the ablation of the expression of a functional protein when crossed to mice with a Cre recombinase gene under the control of a promoter of interest.

Ctnnb$^{loxEx3/wt}$ (Harada, Tamai et al. 1999)

Exon 3 containing Ser/Thr phosphorylation sites for glycogen synthase kinase 3 β (GSK3β) within one Ctnnb allele of these mice is flanked by loxP sequences. Crossing of Ctnnb$^{loxEx3/wt}$ with villin-CreER^{T2} mice results in the expression of a truncated β-catenin protein in IEC, which is prevented from degradation and accumulates in the cytoplasm.

Iκbα$^{F/F}$ (Rupec, Poujol et al. 1999)

A targeting construct was designed inserting loxP sites into the Ikba locus. Crossing these mice to mice containing a Cre recombinase gene under the control of a promoter of interest results in the Cre-mediated deletion of the promoter region containing essential regulatory NF-κB binding sites, the core promoter, and the first two exons of Ikba.

IKKb$^{F/F}$ (Chen, Egan et al. 2003)

A targeting construct was generated by inserting 2 loxP sites flanking exon 3 of the Ikbkb gene, encoding for the IKKβ activation loop. Crossing these mice to mice containing a Cre recombinase gene under the control of a promoter of interest results in the Cre-mediated excision of exon 3 and leads to the ablation of the expression of a functional IKKβ protein.

Lgr5-EGFP-IRES-creER^{T2} (Barker, van Es et al. 2007)

The EGFP-IRES-creERT2 targeting construct was designed by inserting an enhanced green fluorescent protein sequence (EGFP), an internal ribosome entry site (IRES), a CreERT2 fusion gene, a polyA signal, and a loxP-flanked neo cassette into the first ATG codon of the targeted gene. While homozygous mice are not viable, heterozygous Lgr5-EGFP-IRES-CreERT2 mice are viable and fertile. Above described "knock-in" allele abolishes Lgr5 gene function and expresses EGFP and a tamoxifen inducible CreER^{T2} fusion protein from the Lgr5 promoter/enhancer elements. Crossing these mice to mice with a loxP flanked sequence of interest results in recombination and excision of the targeted sequence upon administration of tamoxifen.

LSL-K-ras^{G12D} (Jackson, Willis et al. 2001)

A targeting vector was designed to place a G12D point mutation in exon 1 of the Kras gene and a loxP-flanked STOP element in intron 1, upstream of the mutation. Crossing LSL-K-ras^{G12D} mice to with a Cre recombinase gene under the control of a promoter of interest leads to excision of the stop cassette allowing expression of oncogenic K-Ras in the tissue of interest.

LysM-Cre (Clausen, Burkhardt et al. 1999)

A targeting vector containing a FRT-flanked neo cassette, herpes simplex virus thymidine kinase (TK) genes and NLS -Cre cDNA, was inserted into the endogenous ATG-start site within exon 1 of the Lyzs gene resulting in expression of Cre recombinase from the endogenous Lyzs locus in myeloid cells in mice. When crossed with mice containing loxP site flanked sequence of interest, Cre-mediated recombination results in deletion of the targeted sequence in the myeloid cell lineage, including monocytes, mature macrophages, and granulocytes.

RelA$^{F/F}$ (Algul, Treiber et al. 2007)

A targeting vector was constructed to insert a modified loxP site and the selection marker genes PGK-neo and TK into the Rela genomic locus. Two of the loxP sites flank neo, and the third is located between exons 10 and 11 of the Rela gene. The floxed fragment of Rela contains exons 7–10, which encode a part of the Rel homology domain and the nuclear localization site resulting in the ablation of the expression of a functional protein when crossed to mice with a Cre recombinase gene under the control of a promoter of interest.

Rosa26R-tdTomato (Luche, Weber et al. 2007)

The Rosa-CAG-LSL-tdTomato-WPRE targeting vector was designed by inserting the following elements between exons 1 and 2 of the Gt(ROSA)26Sor locus: a CAG promoter, a FRT site, a loxP-flanked STOP cassette, a tdTomato sequence, a WPRE element to enhance the mRNA transcript stability, a polyA signal, and an attB/attP-flanked neo cassette. Crossing these mice to mice with a Cre recombinase gene under the control of a promoter of interest TdTomato is expressed following Cre-mediated recombination and excision of the loxP flanked STOP cassette.

Tnf$^{-/-}$ (Pasparakis, Alexopoulou et al. 1996)

A targeting vector was constructed by replacing 40 bp of the 5' UTR, all the coding region, including the ATG translation initiation codon, of the first exon and part of the first intron of the Tnf gene with a neomycin cassette in order to generate TNF-deficient mice.

Tp53$^{F/F}$ (Jonkers, Meuwissen et al. 2001)

In these mice exons 2-10 of the Tp53 gene are flanked by loxP sites. When crossed to mice with a Cre recombinase gene under the control of a promoter of interest, expression of p53 is abolished.

Villin-Cre (Madison, Dunbar et al. 2002)

Mice are heterozygous for the transgene expressing Cre recombinase controlled by the mouse villin promoter. Cre recombinase recombines genes flanked by loxP sequences. Crossing of Villin-Cre mice with mice containing a loxP-flanked gene of interest leads to tissue-specific deletion of the targeted sequence.

Villin-Cre ER^{T2} (el Marjou, Janssen et al. 2004)

In these mice a mutated ligand binding domain of the human estrogen receptor is fused to the Cre recombinase transgene leading to induction of Cre expression under the villin promoter only in the presence of tamoxifen. Crossing of Villin-Cre ER^{T2} mice with mice containing a loxP-flanked sequence of interest leads to a spatiotemporal tissue-specific deletion of the targeted sequence upon administration of tamoxifen.

Xbp1s-creER^{T2} modified from (Iwawaki, Akai et al. 2004)

Mice were generated by replacing the coding sequence for the GFP variant venus fused to XBP1 in a pCAX-F-XBP1ΔDBD-venus plasmid (Iwawaki et al., 2004) with the sequence encoding a tamoxifen inducible Cre recombinase under control of the CMV-immediate early promoter. Cre expression is induced upon physiologic splicing of XBP1. Crossing these mice to mice containing a loxP-flanked sequence of interest leads to a deletion of the targeted sequence in all cells being subject to XPB1 slicing.

2.1.2 Genotyping

For genotyping of mice tail samples were lysed overnight at 60°C in 95 μl tail lysis buffer supplemented with 5 μl Proteinase K (Qiagen). The enzymatic digestion was stopped by heat inactivation at 95°C for 10 min. Samples were diluted 1:10 with distilled water and centrifuged for 10 min at 13200 rpm. Supernatants were used for polymerase chain reaction (PCR).

Common PCR-conditions:	An initial denaturation period at 94°C for 5 min was followed by an extension step applying diverse temperatures and an indicated number of cycles for respective genes and a final elongation step for 10 min at 72°C

General PCR reaction mix:

10x PCR buffer (Invitrogen)	2 µl
50 mM $MgCl_2$ (Invitrogen)	0,8 µl
100 mM dNTP Mix (Invitrogen)	0,4 µl
20 pMol Forward Primer	0,5 µl
20 pMol Reverse Primer	0,5 µl
Taq Polymerase (5U/µl) (Invitrogen and self produced)	0,15 µl
DNA	1,5 µl
H_2O	14,15 µl

Tail lysis buffer

Tris/HCl	1,5 M
NaCl	200 mM
SDS	0,2 %
EDTA	5 mM

APC$^{fl/fl}$ 95°C 30 s
60°C 30 s
72°C 60 s
30 cycles
F 5'-GTT CTG TAT CAT GGA AAG ATA GGT GGT C-3'
R 5'-CAC TCA AAA CGC TTT TGA GGG TTG-3'

Ctnnb 94°C 30 s
58°C 30 s
72°C 30 s
35 cycles
wt F 5´- TTC CCA GTC CTT CAC GCA AG - 3´
R 5' - GCA AGT TCC GCG TCA TCC T - 3'

floxed 1,5 mM MgCl2
F 5'-TTC CCA GTC CTT CAC GCA AG -3'
R 5'- CTG AAT GAA CTG CAG GAC GA - 3'

Cre	94°C 30 s	
	58°C 30 s	
	72°C 30 s	
	35 cycles	
	F	5'-ACC TGA AGA TGT TCG CGA TTA TCT-3'
	R	5'-ACC GTC AGT ACG TGA GAT ATC TT-3'
Ikba	94°C 30 s	
	58°C 30 s	
	72°C 30 s	
	35 cycles	
	F	5´- CCA AGC AGA GAC GTG TAT TTC T - 3´
	R	5´- TCC AGA CAG TAA GGG CCA GGT - 3´
Ikbkb	94°C 30 s	
	58°C 30 s	
	72°C 30 s	
	35 cycles	
	F	5´-CAC AGT GCC CAC ATT ATT TAG ATA-3´
	R	5´- GTC TTC AAC CTC CCA AGC CTT - 3´

K-Ras		94°C 30 s
		56°C 60 s
		72°C 60 s
		35 cycles
	F	5´- CCA TGG CTT GAG TAA GTC TGC G - 3´
	R	5´- CGC AGA CTG TAG AGC AGC G - 3´
Lgr5-EGFP-cre		94°C 30 s
		66°C 60 s
		72°C 30 s
		36 cycles
Lgr5 wt F		5'-CTG CTC TCT GCT CCC AGT CT-3'
	R	5'-ATA CCC CAT CCC TTT TGA GC-3'
Lgr5-GFP F		5'-CTG CTC TCT GCT CCC AGT CT-3'
	R	5'-GAA CTT CAG GGT CAG CTT GC-3'
Tp53		94°C 30 s
		58°C 30 s
		72°C 30 s
		35 cycles
	F	5´- CAC AAA AAC AGG TTA AAC CAG - 3´
	R	5´- AGC ACA TAG GAG GCA GAG AC - 3´

RelA		94°C 30 s
		58°C 30 s
		72°C 30 s
		35 cycles
	F	5´- GAG CGC ATG CCT AGC ACC AG - 3´
	R	5´- GTG CAC TGC ATG AGT GCA G - 3´
tdtomato		94°C 60 s
		61°C 30 s
		72°C 30 s
		35 cycles
Wt F		5'-AAG GGA GCT GCA GTG GAG TA-3'
	R	5'-CCG AAA ATC TGT GGG AAG TC-3'
Mut F		5'-GGC ATT AAA GCA GCG TAT CC-3'
	R	5'-CTG TTC CTG TAC GGC ATG G-3'
Tnf		94°C 30 s
		62°C 60 s
		72°C 60 s
		35 cycles
Wt F		5´- TAG CCA GGA GGG AGA ACA GA - 3´
	R	5´- AGT GCC TCT TCT GCC AGT TC - 3´
Mut F		5´- TAG CCA GGA GGG AGA ACA GA - 3´
	R	5´- CGT TGG CTA CCC GTG ATA TT - 3´

2.1.3 AOM administration

In order to induce colonic tumor formation mice were injected with AOM (Sigma) intraperitoneally (i.p.) at a dose of 10 mg/kg bodyweight once a week for 6 weeks. AOM was prepared in sterile 0,9 % sodium chloride up to a final concentration of 0,5 mg/ml.

2.1.4 Tamoxifen administration

In order to induce Cre expression in Cre-ER^{T2} mice 1 mg tamoxifen (Sigma) dissolved in 100 μl pure ethanol mixed with sunflower oil (20% v/v) was orally gavaged once per day for 5 days.

2.1.5 Bone marrow transplantation

In order to deplete the bone marrow, mice were lethally irradiated (9 Gy). Bone marrow from donor mice was isolated in sterile PBS. For adoptive transfer 2-3*10^{6} cells were injected into the tail vein of irradiated mice. The transplanted animals were treated with antibiotics supplemented in the drinking water (1 mg/ml Ciprobay (Bayer)) for two weeks. 4 weeks after the bone marrow transplantation mice were regarded as reconstituted and were challenged with azoxymethane.

2.1.6 FITC-dextran intestinal permeability test

To measure intestinal barrier permeability, non-charged FITC-dextran MW 4000 (Sigma) was prepared at 80 mg/mL in PBS. 4h prior measurement mice were orally gavaged with 60 mg FITC-dextran solution per 100g of body weight. FITC-dextran is only enabled to pass the intestinal barrier in case of a barrier defect. Serum was collected and the serum FITC-dextran level was measured at 485 nm excitation and 510 nm emission wavelength using a fluorometer (BMG Labtech Fluostar Orange).

2.1.7 Depletion of intestinal microflora

To deplete the intestinal microflora mice were treated for two weeks with an antibiotic cocktail in the drinking water containing ampicillin (0.22 g/l), vancomycin (0.1 g/l), neomycin (0.214 g/l) and metronidazole (0.213 g/l). The microflora depletion was confirmed by plating stool samples on Columbia blood agar plates.

2.1.8 Mini endoscopy and confocal laser scanning microscopy (clsm)

In order to monitor distal colorectal tumor growth mice were anesthesized by i.p. injection of MMF adjusted to the body weight (Midazolame (5 mg/g),Medetomidine (0.5 mg/g), Fentamyl (0.05 mg/g) and mini endoscopy was performed using a mouse mini endoscopy system (Karl Storz, Germany). For blood vessel detection mice were anesthesized and injected with 100 µl fluorescein (1%) intravenously (i.v.). A confocal miniprobe (Mauna Kea Technologies, France) was used simultaneously to the mini endoscopy system and video sequences (each 20s, 12 frames/s) were recorded within 10 minutes after i.v. fluorescein injection. Vessel length and vessel area of a minimum of 10 images per tumor were quantified using Cellvizio software.

2.1.9 Sacrifice of mice

1,5 h before sacrifice mice were injected i.p. with 75 mg/kg bromodesoxyuridine (BrdU, Sigma) dissolved in PBS. BrdU is a nucleotide analogue of the base thymidine and is incorporated in the DNA instead of thymidine during cell proliferation. The incorporation of BrdU by proliferating cells can be detected immunohistochemically. After sacrifice colon, small intestine and organs were removed. The different parts of the intestine were flushed with PBS to remove feces and cut open longitudinally. For subsequent histological analysis a "swiss roll" (Moolenbeek and Ruitenberg 1981) was prepared from the different intestinal parts and stored in 4% paraformaldehyde (Electron Microscopy Science) overnight besides other tissues intended for histology. The next day tissues were dehydrated (Leica ASP 300 S) and embedded in paraffin. For further molecular biological analysis tissue pieces of intestinal mucosa were snap frozen in liquid nitrogen and stored at -80°C.

2.1.10 Intestinal epithelial cell isolation

To isolate intestinal epithelial cells (IEC) the intestine was cut into small pieces and incubated in 1xHBSS (Invitrogen) supplemented with 30 mM EDTA (Fluka) for 10 min at 37°C gently shaking. The cell suspension was vortexed for 30 s and incubated on ice. The supernatant including detached epithelial cells was transferred to a new falcon tube and spun down at 1500 rpm for 10 min at 4 °C. The epithelial cell pellet was washed in PBS, transferred to Eppendorf tubes and centrifuged at 5000 rpm for 5 min at 4°C. The supernatants were discarded and the pellets were snap frozen in liquid nitrogen and stored at -80°C.

2.1.11 Villus isolation and propagation

In order to cultivate small intestinal villi *ex vivo* intestines were washed with PBS and opened longitudinally. Villi were removed mechanically using a glass coverslip, washed in PBS and centrifuged at 100 xg for 3 min to separate villi from single cells. 100-150 villi were mixed with 50 µl of Matrigel (BD Bioscence) and plated in 24-well plates in Advanced DMEM/F12 supplemented with growth factors EGF (50 ng/ml, Peprotech) and Noggin (100 ng/ml, Peprotech). Wildtype mice derived villi were cultured with R-spondin (500 ng/ml, R&D System) additionally. Villi were feeded with freshly added growth factors every day. After 1 week, the villi were removed from the Matrigel, washed in fresh medium, centrifuged at 100g for 3 min and plated in fresh Matrigel. For cell sorting, villi were dissociated with TryPLe (Invitrogen) including DNase I for 10 min at 37°C. The cells were passed through a cell strainer with a pore size of 40 µm and GFP+ and GFP- cells were sorted by flow cytometry. Single viable cells were gated by negative staining for Propidium Iodide (PI). For transplantation experiments 50 spheres (containing around 100 cells/sphere) were suspended in 100 µL Matrigel and injected subcutaneously (s.c.) into 6-week-old female athymic (CD1) mice.

2.1.12 Organoid culture

In order to cultivate intestinal crypts *ex vivo* intestines were washed with PBS and opened longitudinally. The villi were mechanically removed using a glass coverslip and intestinal crypts were collected in PBS supplemented with 5mM EDTA. 500 crypts were plated in matrigel and minimal growth medium was added containing 100ng/ml Noggin (Peprotech), 1µg/ml R-Spondin (R&D Systems), 50µg/ml EGF

(Peprotech). For complete single cell medium 50μg/ml Jagged-1 (R&D Systems) was added (Sato et al., 2009). The formation of organoids was assessed after five days.

2.1.13 Bacterial endotoxin test

In order to measure the endotoxin serum level, serum was collected from the hepatic portal vein in the moment of sacrifice. LPS serum level was determined using the endpoint chromogenic Limulus Amebocyte Lysate assay (LONZA) according to the manufacturer's instructions. Gram-negative bacterial endotoxin catalyzes the activation of a proenzyme in the Limulus Amebocyte Lysate (LAL). The initial rate of activation is determined by the concentration of endotoxin present in the serum. The activated enzyme catalyzes the splitting of p-nitroaniline (pNA) from a colorless synthetic substrate, producing a yellow color, which is measured photometrically at 405-410 nm after the reaction is stopped with a stop reagent.

2.2 Human Samples

Human tumor samples were collected within the first 30 minutes after resection. The tumors were macroscopically dissected by an experienced pathologist, snap frozen and stored in liquid nitrogen. Before molecular analysis, the tumor stage was confirmed and tumor content (at least 70%) was determined by hematoxylin-eosin staining.

2.3 Histology

2.3.1 Haematoxylin & Eosin (H&E) staining

For general histological evaluation of tissues, paraffin embedded tissues were cut in 3 μm slices and dried on superfrost glass slides (Thermo

Scientific). The paraffin cuts were deparaffinized for 10 min in xylol (X-TRA Solv, Medite) and rehydrated for 2 minutes each in descending dilutions of ethanol (100%, 96%, 80%, 70%, 50%). The tissues slides were washed in PBS and cell nuclei were stained for 1 min in a ready-to-use haematoxylin solution (Vector Laboratories) and residual staining solution was washed off in running distilled water. In order to stain eosinophilic structures and the cytoplasm tissue slides were stained for 10 s in a 3% eosin (Sigma) solution (acidified with 10 drops acetic acid per 100 ml) and residual staining solution was washed off in distilled water. The tissue was dehydrated in ascending dilutions of ethanol (50%, 70%, 80%, 96%, 100%) for 1 min each and finally incubated in xylol for 5 min. The tissue slides were air dried and preserved in mounting medium (Vector Laboratories) covered by a glass cover slip.

2.3.2 Alcian Blue staining

In order to stain acidic mucosubstances Alcian Blue staining is used. Paraffin tissues samples were deparaffinized and rehydrated as described for H&E staining. Afterwards, tissue slides were incubated for 20 min in a 1% Alcian Blue (Sigma) solution dissolved in 3% acetic acid and washed in distilled water before nuclear counterstaining was done using nuclear fast red solution (Vector Laboratories) for 5 min. The slides were washed in PBS, dehydrated and covered with mounting medium (Vector Laboratories) and a cover slip.

2.3.3 Azure Eosin staining

Azure Eosin staining was performed to stain granule containing Paneth cells. Paraffin tissue samples were deparaffinized and rehydrated as described for H&E staining. After the rehydration, the slides were incubated for 2 hours in a 0,05% azure II (Sigma)/0,01% eosin in water (acidified with 10 drops acetic acid per 100 ml). Afterwards, the slides were washed with distilled water, dehydrated as described and covered with mounting medium (Vector Laboratories) and a cover slip.

2.3.4 Alkaline Phosphatase staining

For alkaline phosphatase staining paraffin sections (3.5µm) were dewaxed and rehydrated as described for H&E staining. Afterwards, the tissue slides were incubated for 2 hrs at RT in nitroblue tetrazolium/5-bromo-4-chloro-3-indolyl phosphate solution (BCIP/NBT ready-to-use solution,Chemicon International), washed with water and nuclei were counterstained with nuclear fast red. The sections were washed with distilled water, dehydrated as described and covered with mounting medium (Vector Laboratories) and a cover slip.

2.3.5 Duolink Proximity Ligation Assay

Protein interactions on paraffin sections were detected by using a Duolink Proximity Ligation Assay (PLA) in situ kit (OLink Bioscience). The principle of the technology is based on two bi-functional probes called PLA probes. Each PLA probe consists of an antibody attached to a unique synthetic oligonucleotide, which acts as a reporter. The oligo-sequence is amplified and the addition of fluorescent probes reveals adjacent proteins. Tissue paraffin sections were dewaxed and rehydrated as described for H&E staining. Ligation Assay in situ kit was used according to the manufacturer's instructions.

2.3.6 Fluorescence in situ hybridization (FISH)

In order to detect and visualize bacteria along the intestinal epithelium fluorescence in situ hybridization was performed using a 5' FITC-labeled universal eubacteria probe (EUB 338: 5'GCTGCCTCCCGTAGGAGT-3') or a Cy3 labeled control probe (NON 338: 5'-CGACGGAGGGCATCCTCA-3'). Probe EUB 338 is complementary to a portion of the 16S rRNA gene conserved in the domain Bacteria (Amann et al., 1990). Freshly prepared 3-5 µm paraffin sections were deparaffinized in Xylol and incubated for 10 minutes in 100% EtOH. The bacterial probes were diluted to a final concentration of 1 ng/ µL in prewarmed hybridization buffer (0.9 M NaCl, 20 mM Tris/HCl, pH 7.3, and 0.1% SDS) and the hybridization was performed at 50°C overnight. Afterwards, the hybridized tissue sections were washed 3 times for 15 min in prewarmed hybridization buffer, rinsed in distilled water and mounted with DAPI containing medium (Invitrogen).

2.3.7 Immunohistochemical analysis

For immunhistochemical analysis parraffin tissue blocks were cut and prepared as described for H&E staining. After dehydration slides were treated for 10 min with with 3% H_2O_2 (Sigma) in order to quench endogenous tissue peroxidases. For retrieving antigens the tissue sections were boiled for 20 min in a microwave in antigen unmasking solution (Vector Laboratories). After cooling down tissue sections were washed in PBS and blocked for 30 min using 3% BSA (Sigma)/PBS supplemented with avidin-block (2 drops per ml, Vector) to block unspecific binding sites for antibodies. Tissue sections were incubated with the first antibody against the epitope of interest diluted in 3% BSA/PBS plus biotin-block (2 drops per ml, Vector Laboratories) over night at 4 °C (respective dilutions are indicated in table 1). The next day, sections were washed 3 times for 5 min in PBS shaking. The secondary antibody conjugated with Biotin (Vector Laboratories) was diluted 1:1000 in 3% BSA/PBS for incubation with the tissue sections for 30 min. An ABC complex solution consisting of avidin dehydroxygenase and biotinylated horseradish peroxidase (Vector Laboratories) was prepared by adding 2 drops of each solution A & B to 5 mL PBS and incubated for 30 min at 4°C prior to use. After washing with PBS the tissue slides were incubated for 30 min with ABC complex solution. For the DAB (3,3'-diaminobenzidine) color reaction, 2 drops of buffer were mixed with 4 drops of DAB and 2 drops of peroxidase (DAB Kit, Vector Laboratories) in 5 ml of distilled water. The staining solution was applied to the tissue slides until the staining for the target of interest was appropriate. The reaction was stopped in distilled water. Nuclei were counterstained with haematoxylin for 1 min, washed with distilled water and dehydrated as described for H&E staining.

Antibody	Company	Catalogue #	Working dilution
Ascl2	Aviva Systems Biology	QC6671	1:200
b-catenin	Santa Cruz Biotechnology	SC-1496	1:400
BrdU	AbD Serotec	MCA 2060	1:400
c-myc	Santa Cruz Biotechnology	SC-788	1:200
cleaved caspase 3	Cell Signaling	9661	1:400
Cxcl1	R&D Systems	MAB453	1:200
E-Cadherin	Becton Dickinson	610182	1:500
EphB3	R&D Systems	AF432	1:50
F4/80	Caltag	MF48000	1:100
Gr-1	eBiosciences	12-5931-82	1:200

Occludin	Invitrogen	711500	1:100
p65	Neo-Markers	RB-1638	1:750
phospho-Histone H2A.X	Cell Signaling	2577	1:200
Sox9	Chemicon Millipore	AB5535	1:200
Twist	Abcam	49254	1:500
VE-Cadherin	Santa Cruz Biotechnology	SC-6458	1:100
Vimentin	Santa Cruz Biotechnology	SC-7557	1:500

Table 1: Antibodies used for immunohistochemical analyses

2.3.8 Digoxigenin-labeling of in situ hybridization probes

The plasmids containing the DNA sequence of interest were designed from I.M.A.G.E clones or FANTOM clones containing the 3'UTR sequences of the respective genes and were kindly provided by Hans Clevers (see table 2). 10 mg of the plasmid DNA was linearized with 30 U of appropriate restriction enzyme for 3h at 37°C. The DNA was purified using a DNA purification kit (Gel extraction kit, Qiagen) and eluted with 10 mL of RNAse free water. The *in vitro* transcription reaction including 2 mg of linearized DNA, 1x transcription buffer (Roche), 10 mM DTT, 1x Dig RNA labeling mix (Roche), 40 U RNAse inhibitor (Roche), 40 U RNA polymerase (T3 or T7, Roche) was performed for more than 2h at 37°C. Afterwards DNA was digested by adding 3U of DNAse I (Qiagen) and incubation for 15 min at 37°C. The RNA was purified by using an RNeasy kit (Qiagen) and eluted in 50 ml of RNAse free water. RNA purification was tested on a denaturing 1% agarose gel. An equal volume of RNAse/DNAse free formamide (Sigma) was added to the RNA probe and stored at -80°C.

	Vector	Restriction enzyme	RNA polymerase	Fragment size (bp)
Mouse Lgr5	pBS-SK+	Spe I	T7	940
Mouse Rnf43	pCMV-Sport6	EcoR I	T7	1630
Human Olfm4	pCR4-TOPO	Hind III	T3	1191

Table 2: in situ probe information

2.3.9 In situ hybridization

In order to detect transcripts of stem cell markers on tissue slides, in situ hybridization was performed. Freshly prepared paraffin sections of 8 μm thickness were incubated at 70 °C overnight, dewaxed and rehydrated as described for H&E staining. Afterwards the sections were treated with 0.2 M HCl for 15 min at room temperature and incubated with proteinase K solution (PBS incl. 30 mg/mL Proteinase K (Qiagen)) for 20 min at 37 °C. Then, the slides were rinsed in 0.2% (w/v) glycine/PBS, washed twice with PBS and postfixed in 4% PFA for 10 min at room temperature. Afterwards, the sections were washed with PBS, treated twice with acetic anhydride solution for 5 min each, washed again with PBS and rinsed in 5x SSC pH 4.5. For prehybridization the slides were placed in a box humidified with 5xSSC/50% formamide and 400 mL hybridization solution was applied to each slide. The sections were incubated for at least 1h at 68°C. The hybridization was carried out for 72h at 68°C after 3 mL of specific digoxigenin labeled probe diluted in 100 mL hybridization buffer was applied to the slides. After the hybridization the slides were rinsed twice in 2x SSC pH 4.5 and washed three times in 50% formamide/2xSSC pH 4.5 for 25 min each at 65 °C.

After washing 5x in TBST (TBS incl. 0.1% Tween 20) the sections were placed in a box humidified with TBST, blocked for 30 min at room temperature in 2% blocking solution (blocking powder (Roche) in TBST) before addition of alkaline phosphatase-conjugated anti-digoxigenin antibody (1:400 in blocking solution, Roche) for incubation overnight at 4°C. The next day, the tissues were washed 5x in TBST, 2x in NTM buffer and incubated overnight at room temperature with nitroblue tetrazolium/5-bromo-4-chloro-3-indolyl phosphate solution (Roche, 1 tablet/10 mL distilled water) for histological detection. Finally the slides were washed in PBS, dehydrated as described for H&E staining and mounted with cover slips.

All buffers were prepared with DEPC water.

DEPC water
  1 mL   DEPC (Sigma)
  1 L   Distilled water

After preparation DEPC water was incubated at room temperature over night and autoclaved before use.

Acetic Anhydride solution
  50 mL   DEPC water
  670 mL   Triethanolamin (Roth)
  5 drops 37% HCl (Merck)
  300 mL   Acetic Anhydride (Roth)

SSC (20x) pH 4.5
  175 g   NaCl (Sigma)
  88 g   Sodium citrate (Sigma)
  1 L   DEPC water

Hybridization solution stock
- 5x SSC
- 5 mM EDTA
- 50 % (v/v) Formamide (Roth)
- 0.05 % (w/v) CHAPS (Sigma)

Hybridization working solution
- Hybridization stock solution +
- 2% (w/v) Blocking powder (Roche)
- 50 µg/mL Yeast total RNA
- 50 µg/mL Heparin

TBST (1x)
- 100 mM Tris pH 7.5
- 150 mM NaCl
- 0.01% (v/v) Tween 20

NTM buffer
- 100 mM Tris pH 9.5
- 100 mM NaCl
- 50 mM $MgCl_2$

2.3.10 TUNEL staining

In order to detect and quantify programmed cell death TUNEL staining was performed, based on the fluorescent labeling of DNA strand breaks. Cleavage of genomic DNA during apoptosis may yield double stranded as well as single strand breaks ("nicks"), which can be identified by marking free 3'-OH termini with fluorescently labeled dUTP in an enzymatic reaction by terminal deoxynucleotidyl transferase. The TUNEL reaction was performed according to the manufacturer's instructions of the commercial ApoAlert DNA-Fragmentation Assay Kit (Clontech). Paraffin sections were dewaxed and rehydrated as described for H&E staining. Samples were incubated for 5 min with a 0,85%

sodium chloride solution and washed with PBS. Subsequently, the tissue sections were postfixed in 4% paraformaldehyde for 15 min, washed again and incubated for 5 min with a 20 µg/ml proteinase K solution. The samples were washed 3 times with PBS and then incubated with the equilibration buffer for 15 min, followed by the application of the enzyme/nucleotide mix in equilibration buffer (30 µl equilibration buffer, 3 µl nucleotide mix, 0,33 µl TdT enzyme per slide). The labeling was accomplished at 37°C for 60 min protected from light. The enzymatic reaction was terminated by incubation in 2x SCC buffer for 15 min at room temperature in the dark and sections were washed twice with PBS. The sections were covered with DAPI mounting medium (ProLong Gold, Invitrogen) and stored at 4°C in the dark.

2.3.11 Tissue hypoxia detection

For immunohistochemical detection of tissue hypoxia a Hypoxyprobe™-1 Plus Kit (Chemicon International, HP2-100) was used and performed according to manufacturer's instructions. 1 hour before sacrificing the mice 60 mg/kg body weight of Pimonidazole Hydrochloride was injected i.p. In hypoxic tissues protein adducts of reductively- activated pimonidazole can be visualized by peroxidase based immunohistochemistry. Formalin-fixed paraffin embedded tissues were deparaffinized and rehydrated as described for H&E staining. Afterwards, endogenous tissue peroxidases were quenched with 3% H_2O_2 (Sigma) for 10 min and antigens were retrieved as described for general immunohistochemistry stainings. The tissues were blocked with 5% BSA/PBS blocking reagent and incubated for 30 min with a primary FITC-conjugated monoclonal antibody (diluted 1:600, Chemicon Int.) directed against pimonidazole protein adducts. The slides were washed 3x 5min in PBS and incubated for another 30 min with a secondary mouse anti-FITC monoclonal antibody (diluted 1:50, Chemicon Int.) conjugated to HRP. The tissue sections were washed in PBS and DAB color reaction was carried out as described for general immunohistochemistry stainings. Nuclei were counterstained with haematoxylin for 1 min, the slides were dehydrated as described above and covered with mounting medium (Vector Laboratories) and a cover slip.

2.4 RNA/DNA analysis

2.4.1 RNA Isolation

For isolation of total RNA from animal tissues an RNeasy Mini Kit (Qiagen) was used and performed according to the manufacturer's instructions. Tissues were lysed in 600 mL RLT buffer supplemented with 1% β-mercaptoethanol. The tissues were lysed using a tissue homogenizer (Polytron PT 1200 E) and were additionally applied to a QIAshredder column (Qiagen). The flow-through was taken for RNA isolation. RNA was eluted in 30 µl of RNase-free water stored at -80°C until further use.

2.4.2 cDNA Synthesis

For cDNA synthesis, the concentration and the purity of the RNA was determined by a Nanodrop spectrophotometer (Thermo scientific). 100 ng -1 µg of RNA in a final volume of 11 µl (filled up with RNase-free water) was incubated with 1 µl of OligodT (50 µM, Invitrogen) and 1 µl of dNTP-mix (10 mM each, Invitrogen) for 5 min at 65°C. Then, the reaction mix was incubated on ice for 1 min and 7 µl of a mastermix was added, containing 4 µl 5x buffer (Invitrogen), 1 µl DTT (0,1 M Invitrogen), 1 µl RNaseOUT (40 units/µl, Invitrogen) and 1 µl SuperscriptII Reverse transcriptase (200 units/µl, Invitrogen). The reverse transcrptase reaction was carried out at 50°C for 60 min. The resulting cDNA was diluted 1:4 with RNase-free water and stored at -20°C.

2.4.3 Real-Time PCR Analysis

The RT-PCR was carried out on a StepOnePlus Real Time PCR cycler (Applied Biosystems) using the indicated primers (see table 3) and the 2x SYBR Green MasterMix (Roche). The primer design was done using Primerexpress 1.0 software. The reaction mix per well contained 12,5 µl of SYBR-Green MasterMix, 9,5 µl of distilled water, 0,5 µl of cDNA and 2,5 µl of the respective primermix (containing 20 mM each: forward and reverse primer). The PCR reaction was performed using standard RT-PCR conditions: 50°C for 2 min, 10 min 95°C, followed by 40 cycles of 95°C for 30 s and 60°C for 1 min. The results were analyzed using the StepOne Software v2.0.2 and normalized according to the expression observed for the house keeping gene cyclophilin using the following equation $2^{(\Delta CT_{Cyclophilin} - \Delta CT_{target gene})}$.

Target	Forward 5´→3´	Reverse 5'→ 3'
Ascl2	GCCCGTGAAGGTGCAAAC	ACAGGAAAAGTGCTCGCGAG
Bax	AAACTGGTGCTCAAGGCCCT	AGCAGCCGCTCACGGAG
Cathepsin B	CCCGACCATTGGACAGATTAGA	CACTGCCCCAAATGCCC
Cathepsin L	GGGTTGTGTGACTCCTGTGAAG	AACCCGATGCGCTAAACG
Cathepsin S	AGCTGCCACGTGTTCAAGGT	TGGCCACTGCTTCTTTCAGG
Ccl 11	CAGAGCTCCACAGCGCTTCT	GGAGCCTGGGTGAGCCA
Ccl 2	CAGCCAGATGCAGTTAACGC	AGCCTACTCATTGGGATCATCTTG
Ccl 21	CATCCCGGCAATCCTGTTC	GCCTTCCTCAGGGTTTGCA
CD 44	CTCCTGGCACTGGCTCTGA	CTGCCCACACCTTCTCCTACTATT
CD68 human	CTTCTCTCATTCCCCTATGGACA	GAAGGACACATTGTACTCCACC
Claudin 1	TTCGCAAAGCACCGGGCAGATACA	GCCACTAATGTCGCCAGACCTGAAA
Claudin 15	GGCTTCCTGGGCCTCTTTC	AGCAGCTTGGCCTTCTTGG
Claudin 2	TGCGACACACAGCACAGGCATCACC	TCAGGAACCAGCGGCGAGTAGAA
Claudin 3	AGCATCATCACGGCGCA	TGCTCTGCACCACGCAGT
Claudin 5	TTAAGGCACGGGTAGCACTCACG	TTAGACATAGTTCTTCTTGTCGTAATCG
Claudin 6	ACTATGCTGCGCCTGCTCTTCTGG	GATATTCGGAGGGTCCCCGAGA
Cxcl1	TATCGCCAATGAGCTGCG	GGATGTTCTTGAGGTGAATCCC
Cxcl10	GAATCCGGAATCTAAGACCATCAA	GTGCGTGGCTTCACTCCAGT
Cxcl2	ATCCAGAGCTTGAGTG	AAGGCAAACTTTTTGA

	TGACGC	CCGCC
Cyclophilin	ATGGTCAACCCCACCGTGT	TTCTGCTGTCTTTGGAACTTTGTC
E-Cadherin	GATTTGAGCCAGCTGCACAG	GGGTGGGAGCCACATCATT
EphB3	ACTTCGCTGGTCATTGCCC	AGCTTGAGTGGTACAGAGACCTCC
Fibronectin 1	AGAGCTTGATCCTGTCTACCTCACA	CAATGGAAGTATCATCAACCTGGTC
Fstl1	CAAGATCTGCGCCAATGTGTT	CGT GGG CTC CCC CTT C
Glut3	TTGGTTTGGACTTTATTCTGGGC	CAAAGCTATCACGGAGATGACG
Igfpb4	AACATCCCAACAACAGCTTCAAC	TTGGCCATATGCTTCTGCAG
IL-11	CTGCACAGATGAGAGACAAATTCC	GAAGCTGCAAAGATCCCAATG
IL-1b	GTGGCTGTGGAGAAGCTGTG	GAAGGTCCACGGGAAAGACAC
Jam A	TCCCTATGCGGACCGAGTC	ATTGTCCTTCCGGGTCACAG
Lgr5	GAGGAAGCGCTACAGAATTTGAGA	GTGGCACGTAGCTGATGTGG
LifR	ATGTGGTCGTGTCTTACTGCCC	CCCCTCCCACTTCATCGG
Mdm2	AATCCTCCCCTTCCATCACACT	GATTTCCACTTTATCTTTCCCCTTATC
Mgmt	CGTGCAGTAGGAGGAGCAATC	GAACCACCCTGTGGCAGG
MMP 10	AAAGGAAGTCAGTTCTGGGCAG	AGTGTGGATCCCCTTTGGGT
MMP 13	ACAAGCAGTTCCAAAGGCTACAA	AGTGATCCAGACCTAGGGAGTGG
MMP 2	CCCCCATGAAGCCTTGTTTA	CTGGAAGCGGAACGGGA
MMP 3	TGGCTCATGCCTATGCACC	ATCCTCTGTCCATCGTTCATCA

MMP 9	CAGCTGGCAGAGGCATACTTG	GCTTCTCTCCCATCATCTGGG
Muc-1	GAGCCAGGACTTCTGGTAGGCT	GGCTTCACCAGGCTTACGTAGT
Muc-2	TCGCCCAAGTCGACACTCA	GCAAATAGCCATAGTACAGTTACACAGC
Noxa	CTCCCAGGAAGGAAGTTCCG	CGAGCGTTTCTCTCATCACATC
Ptgs2	CAGCCAGGCAGCAAATCCT	CTTATACTGGTCAAATCCTGTGCTCA
Puma	ACGACCTCAACGCGCAGT	GTGAGGGTCGGTGTCGATG
Rnf43	TCCACCTCATTCGCCAGC	GAAGGCCCCAACAGATAGGC
Sox9	GCAGACCAGTACCCGCATCT	TCTCGTTCAGCAGCCTCCA
Sucrose isomaltase	CAACCTCGGCAAAACCTTTATAGT	TGCAGCCTCTCTCTACGCAA
Synaptophysin	TTCGTGAAGGTGCTGCAGTG	TCTCCGGTGTAGCTGCCG
Tenascin C	GGCCCCGGCTTGAAGA	GGTGATCAGTGCTGTGGTGTCT
TNF-α	ACTCCAGGCGGTGCCTATG	GAGCGTGGTGGCCCCT
Tnfrsf19	CGCTGGTGAACCGCTTTC	CAGGCAGTCCCCGCAG
Trail	GGATATGGCCTGGCTGTAGA	GTTCCAGCTGCCTTTCTGTC
Twist	GCTGGACTCCAAGATGGCA	AGACGGAGAAGGCGTAGCTG
Versican	ATCAATGGGAAGCAGCTCGT	GGCCACGCCTAGCTTCTG
Vimentin	ATCGACAAGGTGCGCTTCC	TTGCCCTGGCCCTTGA
Zfp503	CCCCTTGAAGCTGAGCGA	CGGGTTTGGAGTAAGGCTTG

Table 3: Real-time primer sequences

2.4.4 Microarray

The Gene expression profiling of intestinal tumors and epithelial cells was performed by probing the Affymetrix Gene ST GeneChip (~ 28.000 genes) with RNA from the respective tissue. The analysis was carried out using the SAM 3.0 software (significance analysis of microarray). In order to test for the enrichment of a NF-κB target gene set overexpressed at the invasive front in human colorectal adenocarcinomas (Horst, Budczies et al. 2009) in transcripts of mouse intestinal tumor tissue or enrichment of the stem cell transcriptome (van der Flier, van Gijn et al. 2009) in transcripts of isolated epithelial cells a gene set enrichment analysis (Subramanian, Tamayo et al. 2005) (GSEA; Broad Institute of MIT and Harvard University (http://www.broad.mit.edu/gsea)) was performed. The use of the GSEA software allows the statistical assessment of an enrichment of signaling pathway signatures in a phenotype of interest. Following parameters were used for the analyses: permutation number 1000; collapse dataset to gene symbols "false". Gene sets smaller than 15 and larger than 500 were excluded.

2.4.5 DNA isolation

In order to isolate DNA from tumor tissues a DNeasy Blood & Tissue Kit (Qiagen) was used according to the manufacturer's instructions. Before isolation, tissue pieces were digested in a Proteinase K containing buffer (Qiagen) at 56 °C over night.

2.4.6 Array comparative genomic hybridization

Array-CGH was carried out according to the manufacturer's instructions using mouse genome CGH 180K microarray kit (Agilent Technologies). 1 µg test DNA and reference DNA was enzymatically labeled with dUTP-Cy5 or dUTP-Cy3. Slides were scanned using a microarray scanner and the images were analyzed using DNA Analytics 4.0 (Agilent Technologies) with the statistical algorithm ADM-2.

2.5 Cloning

2.5.1 Cloning of the CreER^{T2} sequence into the ER stress indicator (ERAI) plasmid

In order to generate a mouse model expressing a tamoxifen inducible Cre recombinase in cells, which are subject to physiological splicing of the ER stress related indicator protein XBP-1, a plasmid construct was generated containing the CreER^{T2} cDNA sequence fused to a XBP-1 sequence behind the 26 nt splice site hence replacing the sequence of the yellow fluorescent protein derivative venus.

The pCAX-F-XBP1delDBD-venus plasmid (Iwawaki, Akai et al. 2004), originally designed as an ER stress indicator (ERAI) plasmid, was digested with the restriction enzymes Bam H I (NEB) and Bgl II (NEB) for 2h at 37 °C to cut out the venus sequence. The restriction of the plasmid was confirmed on a 1% agarose gel. The linearized plasmid fragment without the venus sequence was eluted from the agarose gel using a Gel Extraction Kit (Qiagen). Afterwards, the 5' phosphates were removed from the vector by dephosphorylation with 10 U of calf intestinal phosphatase (CIP, NEB) for 20 min at 37 °C to prevent religation. In order to circumvent a translational reading frame shift in the Cre recombinase sequence in the case of a direct blunt end ligation of the pCAX vector backbone and the CreER^{T2} sequence, an intermediate cloning step was included in which the pCAX vector was ligated to a linker oligonucleotide containing the restriction sites for BglII, EcoRI, SacI and BamHI. Then, the linker containing plasmid was digested with EcoRI and SacI for 2h at 37 °C to linearize the plasmid. The CreER^{T2}

sequence containing plasmid was digested with EcoRI and SacI in the same way. The restriction was confirmed on a 1 % agarose gel. The CreER^{T2} fragment as well as the linearized pCAX vector band were eluted from the agarose gel using a Gel Extraction kit (Qiagen) and both fragments were ligated via the EcoRI and SacI restriction sites. The correct sequence and orientation of the insert was confirmed by sequencing analysis using the following primer: GAAGCCAAGGGGAATGAAGT.

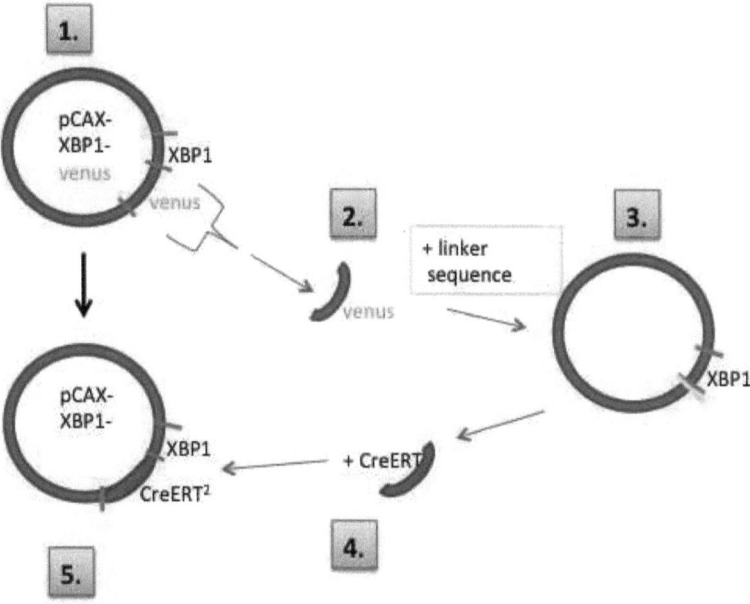

Cloning scheme of the CreER^{T2} sequence insertion into the ERAI plasmid

(1) scheme of the original ERAI plasmid (2) excision of the venus sequence (3) ligation of the pCAX vector with a linker sequence (4) restriction of the linker containing pCAX vector and ligation with the CreER^{T2} sequence (5) pCAX-plasmid containing the CreER^{T2} sequence instead of the venus sequence

2.5.2 Ligation of a linker oligonucleotide into a vector construct

The designed linker oligonucleotides (oligo) were dissolved in distilled water at a concentration of 200 mM. A doublestrand oligo at a concentration of 50 mM each was produced by annealing for 4 min at 95 °C and cooling down for 30 min at room temperature. For ligation with a linearized vector construct a final concentration of 100nM or 200 nM of annealed oligo was used and ligation was performed with 1 U T4 DNA Ligase (Invitrogen) overnight at 4°C.

	For (5'→ 3')	Rev (5'→ 3')
pCAX -linker	GATCTTTGAATTCGAGCTCG	GATCCGAGCTCGAATTCAAA

2.5.3 Ligation

Ligation of DNA constructs was performed overnight at 4°C by using 1 U of T4 Ligase (Invitrogen) in a total volume of 20 mL using a vector-insert molecular ratio of 1:3.

2.5.4 Transformation

The ligated vector construct was transformed by heatshock in XL-1 blue competent bacteria. A 100 mL aliqot of competent bacteria was thawed on ice for 5 min, 2 mL of the ligation was added and incubated on ice for 30 min. The heatshock was performed for 45 sec at 42 °C and the transformed bacteria were immediatly stored on ice for 2 min before adding 700 mL of LB medium. The bacteria were incubated for 1h at 37 °C shaking before the bacterial culture was plated on LB-Agar plates including the appropriate antibiotics. The plates were incubated overnight at 37 °C.

LB medium

                    1% (w/v)   Tryptone (BD)
                    0.5% (w/v) Yeast extract (BD)
                    1% (w/v)   NaCl

2.5.5 Isolation of plasmid DNA from bacteria

Single colonies from transformed bacteria on LB-agar plates were inoculated in 2 ml of LB-broth containing 100 µg/ml ampicillin and incubated overnight while shaking at 37 °C. In order to isolate a plasmid from the bacterial culture a Qiaprepe Miniprep Kit (Qiagen) was used and performed according to the manufacturer's instructions. The DNA concentration was determinded by using NanoDrop (Thermo Scientific).

2.6 Chromatin Immunoprecipitation analysis (ChIP)

For detecting the interaction of a transcription factors with a DNA sequence of interest chromatin immunoprecipitation was performed. IEC were isolated as described above and proteins were cross-linked to DNA with 1% formaldehyde for 10 min at room temperature. Formaldehyde was quenched for 10 min at room temperature by adding glycine (0.125M final concentration). The IEC were washed in PMSF/PBS (0.5 mM final concentration) by centrifugation at 2200 rpm for 5 min at 4°C and lysed in lysis buffer (Active Motif) supplemented with protease inhibitor cocktail (Active motif) for 20 min on ice. The chromatin was fragmented for 5x 20 sec and 30 sec breaks on ice in between each step by using a sonifyer. Afterwards, the chromatin was precleared using 2.5 mg/mL salmon sperm/protein A agarose (Upstate) for 1 h. Chromatin immunoprecipitation was performed overnight rotating at 4°C using 1.5 µg of the respective antibody. The next day, 25 mL Dynabeads Protein G (Invitrogen) were added to the antibody/chromatin solution and incubated for 1h at 4°C. By means of a magnetic bead holder facility bound chromatin complexes were washed twice with icecold ChIP buffer 1 (Active motif), 2x with high salt buffer (50 mM Tris pH 8, 500 mM NaCl, 0.1% SDS, 0.5% Sodium deoxycholate, 1% NP40, 1 mM EDTA), 2x with LiCl buffer (50 mM Tris pH 8, 1 mM EDTA, 250 mM LiCl, 1% NP40, 0.5% Sodium deoxycholate), 2x with ChIP buffer 2 (Active motif) and finally 1x with PBS before precipitates were eluted in TE containing 1% SDS and 150 mM NaCl and incubated over night at 65°C to reverse crosslinking. The next day, Proteinase K was added (1 mg/mL final concentration) and incubated for 1h at 56 °C. The DNA was purified using a QiaAmp DNA Micro Kit (Qiagen) and eluted in 100 mL elution buffer according to the manufacturer's instructions prior to Real-Time PCR. For the RT-PCR reaction 5 mL of DNA were used, 2 mL of 20 mM primermix (20 mM of forward and reverse primer each, s. table 4), 3 mL distilled water and 10 mL 2x SYBR Green mix (Roche). The RT-PCR reaction conditions were applied as described above. The results were analyzed using the StepOne Software v2.0.2 and normalized according to the expression level detected for the input DNA.

Promoter	Forward 5´→3´	Reverse 5'→ 3'
Ascl2	AGGTCAGTGCATTTCCCTTCC	ACCTCTCAGTCCCATCCTTCC
Lgr5	AAGCACCATGAAGCTGGAAGA	GGAGCATAGCGTTGCCGT
Sox9	TCAACCCCGGAGTAGTTTTGC	CTTGCCTCCTGACTGAGTCACA

Table 4: RT-PCR ChIP primer sequences

2.6.1 Sequential ChIP (Re-ChIP)

In order to detect the simultaneous binding of NF-κB and β-catenin on promoter regions of interest two sequential immunoprecipitations (IP) were done by means of a Re-ChIP-it Kit (Active Motif). The chromatin for the first IP was prepared and IP procedure itself was performed as described above. Afterwards, the chromatin was washed in the same manner as described above and eluted in Re-ChIP-it elution buffer (Active Motif). The chromatin was desalted using desalting columns (Active Motif) and the second IP was set up according to the manufacturer's instructions. The next day, the chromatin was eluted, crosslinking was reversed and treated with Proteinase K as described in the kit manual. The RT-PCR experiment and analysis was carried out as described above.

2.7 Protein analysis

2.7.1 Preparation of Protein lysates

In order to extract proteins tissues were lysed in 200 µl ice cold protein lysis buffer by mechanical homogenization with a micro-pistill. Lysates were incubated for 10 min on ice before centrifugation at 13200 rpm at 4°C for 10 min to pellet cell debris. Protein containing supernatants were stored at -80°.

Protein lysis buffer
- 50 mM, pH 7.8 Tris (Roth)
- 250 mM NaCl (Sigma)
- 30 mM EDTA (Sigma)
- 30 mM EGTA (Sigma)
- 25 mM Sodium-pyrophosphate (Sigma)
- 1% Triton-X 100 (Sigma)
- 0.5% NP40 (Sigma)
- 10% Glycerol (Merck)
- 1 mM DTT (Sigma)
- 50 mM β-glycerophosphate (Sigma)
- 25 mM Sodium fluoride (Sigma)
- 5 mM Sodium orthovanadate (Sigma)
- 2 nM PMSF (Sigma)
- 1 tablet of complete-protease inhibitor cocktail tablets (Roche)/ 50 mL

2.7.2 Western Blot analysis

For immuoblot analysis acrylamide gels were prepared with an appropriate acrylamide percentage depending on the size of the proteins to be analyszed (s. table 5). The protein concentration of the samples was measured in a spectrophotometer (Nanodrop, Thermo Scientific) at a wavelength of 595 nm by mixing 2µl of the lysates with 1 ml of 1:5 diluted Bradford protein assay solution (BioRad). A protein standard curve was set up using BSA. 15-50 µg of protein were adjusted to a volume of 24 µl by filling up with protein lysis buffer, and 8 µl of 4x Laemmli buffer was added. The samples were boiled at 95°C for 5 min, cooled down on ice, briefly centrifuged and loaded onto the gel. The gel was run at 120 volt in 1x running buffer.

%	Acrylamide (mL)	Resolving Gel buffer (mL)	Distilled water (mL)	10% APS (µL)	TEMED (µL)
6	1.5	2.5	6	50	5
7	1.7	2.5	5.8	50	5
7.5	1.8	2.5	5.7	50	5
8	2.03	2.5	5.5	50	5
10	2.5	2.5	5	50	5
12	3	2.5	4.4	50	5
15	3.75	2.5	3.65	50	5

Table 5: Acrylamide gel composition

Resolving Gel buffer
        0.5 M, pH 6.8 Tris
        0.4 % (w/v) SDS (Fluka)

Stacking Gel buffer
        1.5 M pH 8.8 Tris
        0.4 % (w/v) SDS (Fluka)

Laemmli buffer
        200 mM, pH 6.8 Tris
        40% (v/v) Glycerol
        8% (w/v) SDS
        0,4% (w/v) Bromophenol blue (Sigma)
        5% (v/v) β-mercaptoethanol (Sigma)

Running buffer (10x)
        9.5 M Glycine (Roth)
        0.25 M Tris
        35 mM SDS

The protein gel transfer was performed using the Mini Trans-Blot Cell system (BioRad) in 1x transfer buffer for 60 min at 400 mA onto a PVDF membrane (Immobilon P, Zefa Laborservice) which has been activated for 30 sec in methanol. After the transfer the membrane was washed in

PBST and incubated for 30 min at room temperature in 3% (w/v) skim milk (Fluka) in PBST to block unspecific binding of antibody. The primary antibody (s. table. 6) was applied onto the membrane at 4°C over night. The next day, the membrane was washed 3 times for 5 min in PBS-T and was incubated with a HRP-labeled secondary antibody (α-rabbit/α-mouse/α-goat, GE Healthcare) in 3% (w/v) skim milk) in PBST for 1 h at room temperature. Afterwards, the membrane was washed again 3 times for 5 min with PBS-T. For protein band detection an ECL solution (Super Signal West Pico or Super Signal West Femto, Thermo Scientific) was applied on the protein side of the membrane for 5 min. The solution was tapped off and the membrane was dried briefly between two Whatman papers and incubated with a X-ray film (Thermo Scientific) for an appropriate time period depending on the signal strength.

Transfer buffer (10x)

        9.5 M   Glycine
        0.25 M Tris

Transfer buffer (1x)

        100 mL 10x Transfer buffer
        200 mL Methanol (Merck)
        700 mL distilled water

PBST

                    PBS (Invitrogen)
    0.1% (v/v) TWEEN 20 (Sigma)

Antibody	Company	Catalogue #	Working dilution
β-actin	Sigma	A4700	1:2000
β-catenin	Santa Cruz Biotechnology	sc-1496	1:500
CBP	Santa Cruz Biotechnology	sc-369	1:500
E-Cadherin	BD	610182	1:500
Ikba	Santa Cruz Biotechnology	sc-371	1:500
p65	Santa Cruz Biotechnology	sc-372	1:1000
phospho-ikba (S32)	Cell Signaling	2859S	1:1000
phospho-p65 (S-276)	Cell Signaling	3037	1:1000
phospho-Stat3 (Y705)	Cell Signaling	9145L	1:1000
Stat3	BD	610190	1:2000
Twist	Abcam	ab49254	1:500

Table 6: Antibodies used for Western blot analyses

2.7.3 DNA Affinity Precipitation Assay (DAPA)

In order to detect the binding strength of β-catenin to consensus Tcf/Lef binding sites a DNA affinity precipitation assays (DAPA) was performed. 150-300 mg of protein lysates, prepared as described above, were incubated for 1.5 h at room temperature with 2 μg of 5' biotin labeled double-stranded oligonucleotides containing two Tcf/Lef binding sites (5'-CCCTTTGATCTTACCCCCTTTGATCTTACC-3') or a scrambled control oligonucleotide (5'-TTTCCCCTTGATACCTTTCCCCTTGATACC-3'). Before, oligonucleotides had been diluted to 10 mM in distilled water, annealed for 10 min at 80°C and cooled down at room temperature. 25 mL of Streptavidin-Agarose beads (Pierce), washed with protein lysis buffer, were added to the protein samples and incubation was continued on a rotator at 4°C overnight. The next day, proteins bound to the beads were washed with protein lysis buffer and boiled in 1x Laemmli buffer at 95°C for 5 min shaking before proteins were detected as described for Western Blot procedure.

2.7.4 EMSA ([γ-^{32}P] ATP radioactively labeled oligonucleotide)

For evaluating the binding activity of NF-κB to its consensus promoter binding site an eletrophoretic mobility shift assay (EMSA) is performed. An oligonucleotide probe containing the NF-κB binding site (5' GGA TCC TCA ACA GAG GGG ACT TTC CGA GGC CA 3') was labeled with [g-^{32}P] ATP for 30 min at 37°C. The probe labeling reaction mix contained 1 ng/mL of annealed oligos (annealing procedure described above for DAPA), 1x polynucleotide kinase buffer (PNK buffer, New England Biolabs), 10 U T4 polynucleotide kinase (NEB) and 50 pmol [g-^{32}P] ATP in a total reaction volume of 20 mL. In order to remove unbound [g-^{32}P] ATP after the reaction, the labeled probe was purified on a pre-spinned sepharose column (G50, GE Healthcare). The protein lysates from intestinal epithelial cells were produced as described above. 10 mg of protein extract was inubated with 1 mL of fresh [g-^{32}P] ATP labeled oligo, 2 mg Poly(dI-dC), 1 mM DTT and 1x EMSA running buffer in a total reaction volume of 20 mL for 30 minutes at room temperature. 2 mL of 10x EMSA loading buffer was added to the binding reaction before it was run on a 5 % native TBE acrylamide gel at 200 V for 1.5 hours in 0.5x TBE running buffer. The protein-DNA complexes were visualized by autoradiography.

EMSA loading buffer (10x)
- 250 mM Tris pH 7.6
- 40% (v/v) Glycerol
- 0.2% (w/v) Bromophenol blue

EMSA running buffer (10x)
- 100 mM Tris pH 7.6
- 500 mM KCl (Sigma)
- 10 mM EDTA
- 50% Glycerol

TBE buffer (5x)
- 500 mM Tris
- 500 mM Boric acid (Sigma)
- 10 mM EDTA

5% native polyacrylamide gel
- 10 mL 5x TBE buffer
- 6.25 mL 40% acrylamide/bis-acrylamide
- 34.5 mL TEMED (Sigma)
- 337 mL 10% (w/v) APS (Merck)
- 33.38 mL Distilled water
- Σ 50 mL

2.7.5 EMSA (3' DY682 infrared marker labeled oligonucleotide)

For evaluating the binding activity of NF-κB in a non-radioactive manner an Odyssey Infrared EMSA Kit (LICOR) was used and performed according to the manufacturer's instructions. 10 μg of protein samples, prepared as described above, were incubated with 1 μM 3' DY682 labeled NF-κB consensus oligo (as indicated above) for 30 min at room temperature protected from light. Afterwards, the samples were run on a 5% native TBE acrylamide gel for 90 min and bands were detected on an Odyssey infrared imaging system (Li-COR biosciences).

2.7.6 Kinase Assay

In order to detect the endogenous kinase activity of a kinase in a total protein lysate a kinase assay was performed. For the first step, immunoprecipitation of the kinase, 15 µl of Sepharose ProteinA beads (GE Healthcare) per sample were incubated with 2 µg of specific antibody (α-IKKγ, BD) and 200-300 µg of total protein lysate overnight at 4°C rotating. The next day, the beads were washed with protein lysis buffer, resuspended in 500 µl 1x kinase assay buffer and incubated for 20 min at 4 °C rotating. Afterwards, the beads samples were resuspended in 15 µl 2x kinase assay buffer and 15 µl of a mastermix was added consisting of 1 µg kinase substrate (GST-ikba (1-54)), 10 mM ATP-solution, 0,5 µl [γ-^{32}P]-ATP (Perkin Elmer) and incubated for 20 min at 37°C. The kinase activity was stopped by adding 7 µl of Laemmli buffer and boiling for 5 min at 95°C. The beads were pelleted by centrifugation at 13000 rpm for 5 min and 20 µl of the sample were loaded on a 10 % acrylamide gel. After the gel run the proteins were blotted on a PVDF membrane as described for western blot analysis. The membrane was exposed to an X-ray film (Kodak BioMax) overnight at -80°C for signal detection.

Kinase Assay buffer (10x)
    0.25 M Hepes pH 7.5
    1.5 M NaCl
    0.25 M β-Glycerophosphate (Sigma)
    0.1 M MgCl2

ATP solution
    10 mM ATP
    100 mM Tris pH 7.5
    50 mM MgCl2
    10 mM DTT

2.8 Cell Culture

2.8.1 Cultivation

Hek293 cells were grown adherent in DMEM (Gibco) including 10% FCS (Gibco) and 1% PenStrep (Gibco) in a 37 °C incubator at 5 % CO_2 air content. Cells were subcultivated 1:10 weekly.

2.8.2 Transfection

In order to transfect Hek293 cells with plasmids containing the protein encoding sequence of interest Lipofectamine (Invitrogen) was used according to the manufacturer's instructions. For the transfection seeded cells are required to have ~50% confluency. The transfection was carried out in 6-Well dishes and cells were covered with 1.5 mL of normal growth medium at the time point of transfection. 1 mg of each vector was diluted in 250 mL of Opti-MEM minimal medium (Gibco). Separately, a 2.5 fold amount of Lipofectamine was diluted in 250 mL of Opti-MEM minimal medium as well. The setup was incubated for 5 min at room temperature. Afterwards, DNA and Lipofectamine solution were combined and incubated for at least 25 min to complex. The DNA-Lipofectamine mix was added to the medium of the cells and incubated overnight (at least 8h) in the incubator. The next day, the transfection medium was replaced by normal growth medium. After 24h cells are considered to be successfully transfected, expressing the sequences of interest and were used for further analysis.

2.8.3 siRNA mediated knockdown

To induce a knockdown of CBP, Hek293 cells were transfected with Lipofectamine as described above along with 120 nM of an ON-

TARGETplus siRNA SMARTpool (Dharmacon RNAi Technologies) targeting CBP or the same amount of a negative control ON-TARGETplus siCONTROL Non- Targeting Control Pool siRNA (Dharmacon RNAi Technologies). After 48h knockdown was confirmed by immunoblot analysis.

2.8.4 Luciferase Assay

In order to assess β-catenin binding activity in cell lysates a Luciferase Assay System (Promega) was applied. Before, cells were transfected as described above with a TOPflash TCF reporter plasmid (Upstate) containing two sets of three copies of the TCF binding site upstream of the Thymidin kinase (TK) minimal promoter and a Luciferase open reading frame. Accordingly, FOPflash containing mutated TCF binding sites was transfected as a negative control. After the transfecion was accomplished, cells were lysed in 100 mL 1x lysis buffer (Promega) and 20 mL Luciferase Assay substrate (Promega) was added shortly before the luciferase activity was measured in a luminometer.

2.9 Statistics

Statistical analysis methods were the standard two-tailed Student's t-test for two data sets and ANOVA followed by Bonferroni/Dunn post hoc tests for multiple data sets using GraphPad Prism 6 software, p-values ≤ 0.05 were considered to be significant. *≤ 0.05; **≤ 0.01; ***≤ 0.001.

3. Results

3.1 The role of NF-κB during tumor initiation

3.1.1 Massive crypt compartment expansion and hyperproliferation of intestinal epithelial cells upon constitutive β-catenin activation promoted by Tnf-α dependent NF-κB activity

In order to study tumor initiation depending on aberrant Wnt signaling, a mouse model displaying a tamoxifen inducible conditional stable expression of β-catenin in intestinal epithelial cells (IEC) was used (villin-creER^{T2}/Ctnnb$^{loxEx3/wt}$, termed β-cat$^{c.a.}$ in the following). After oral application of tamoxifen, Cre dependent recombination of the β-catenin gene was induced in all intestinal epithelial cells. The excision of exon 3 by Cre recombinase resulted in a cytoplasmatically stabilized β-catenin protein due to loss of important phosphorylation sites and therefore resistance to GSK3β-mediated proteasomal degradation (Harada, Tamai et al. 1999). Accumulation of mutated β-catenin thereupon led to constitutively active Wnt-signaling which brought about an almost total loss of differentiated, absorptive enterocytes and a massive expansion of highly proliferative crypt stem cell compartment expressing high levels of the Wnt target c-myc (Fig. 8 A-H). β-cat$^{c.a.}$ mice exhibited marked weight loss and died within 27 days after phenotype induction (Fig. 8 I). Strikingly, intestinal epithelial cells feature enhanced IκB kinase activity (Fig. 8 J) as well as NF-κB binding activity, which was confirmed histologically by nuclear accumulation of p65/RelA within transformed crypt cells. (Fig. 8 K, L, N). In order to elucidate the cause of NF-κB activation, β-cat$^{c.a.}$ mice were treated pharmacologically using etanercept and anakinra which inhibited TNF-α and IL-1β, respectively, as both cytokines are the major upstream activators of NF-κB. While inhibition of IL-1b did not have an effect, blockage of TNF-α reduced NF-κB binding activity, correlating with a significantly prolonged survival in β-cat[c.a.] mice bred with TNF[-/-] mice (Fig. 8 O, P) indicating that NF-κB was primarily activated extrinsically in IEC of β-cat[c.a.] mice by paracrine and/or autocrine secreted TNF-α.

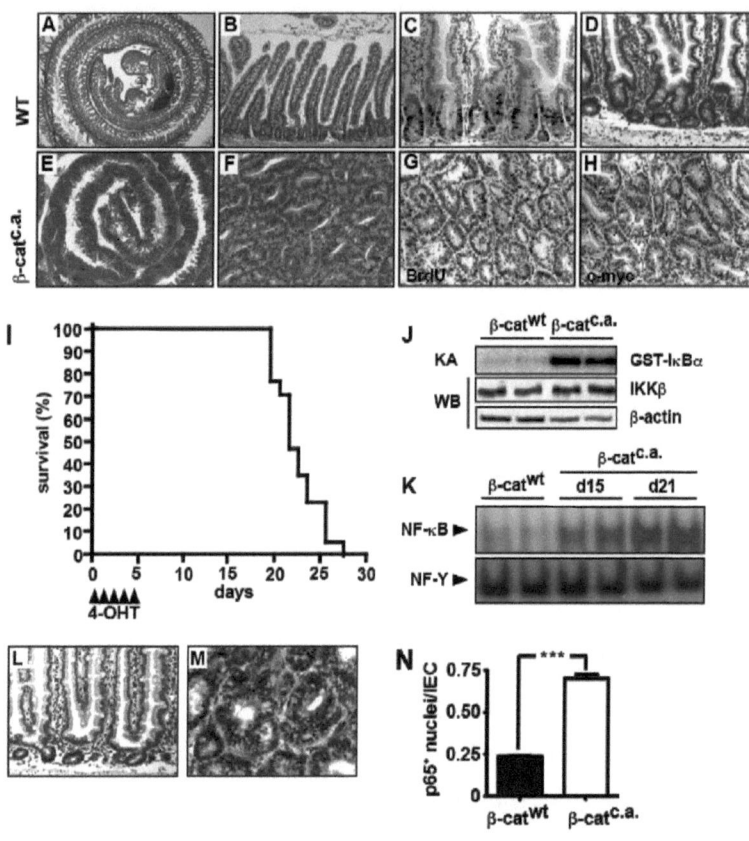

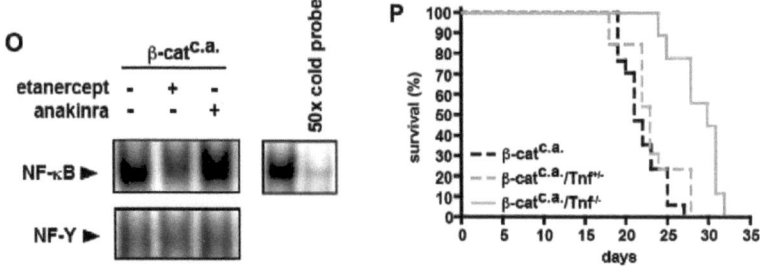

A colored version is available in the electronic edition

Figure 8: Hyperactivation of β-catenin results in crypt stem cell hyperproliferation and NF-κB activation

Histological H&E stained (A,B,E,F) and immunohistochemical (C,D,G,H) stainings of the duodenum from histologically unchanged wildtype (A-D) and tamoxifen induced b-cat$^{c.a.}$ animals showing crypt compartment hyperproliferation and loss of differentiated enterocytes (E,F,G) in line with expression of proliferation stem cell marker c-myc (H). (I) Kaplan-Meier survival curve of β-cat$^{c.a.}$ mice. (J) Kinase Assay shows increased IκB-kinase activity in IEC of β-cat$^{c.a.}$ mice compared to wildtype mice 21 days after tamoxifen administration. (K) EMSA depicting enhanced NF-κB activation in IEC of β-cat$^{c.a.}$ mice after 15 or 21 days of phenotype induction. (L) Immunohistochemistry of RelA/p65 in wildtype duodenum and in (M) β-cat$^{c.a.}$ hyperproliferative duodenum. (N) Quantification of nuclear RelA/p65 cells per cell. Data are mean ± SE; n=3; *** p < 0.0001 by two-tailed Student's t-test (Prism) (O) EMSA: TNF-α inhibitor etanercept but not IL-1β inhibitor anakinra blocks NF-κB activity. Competetive, excessive (50x) addition of unlabeled oligo confirmed specificity. (P) Kaplan-Meier survival curve of β-cat$^{c.a.}$/Tnf$^{-/-}$ mutant mice (solid line; n=9) compared to β-cat$^{c.a.}$/Tnf$^{+/-}$ mice (light dashed line; n=13; p< 0.0001 by log rank test); survival of β-cat$^{c.a.}$ mice is shown as a comparison (black dashed line).

3.1.2 NF-κB triggers the initiation of adenomatous cell transformation by modulating Wnt-dependent intestinal stem cell gene expression

In order to specifically investigate the causal role of NF-κB on the phenotype of β-cat$^{c.a.}$ mice, p65 was deleted in IEC by crossing β-cat$^{c.a.}$ mice to floxed RelA mice (Algul, Treiber et al. 2007) (mice are termed β-cat$^{c.a.}$/RelA^{ΔIEC} hereafter). β-cat$^{c.a.}$/RelA^{ΔIEC} displayed a significantly increased survival by around 50 % compared to β-cat$^{c.a.}$ mice, which was even more distinct than by loss of TNF-α in all cells, suggesting also other upstream effects to activate the NF-κB pathway in this case (Fig. 9A).

All mice were examined on day 15 after tamoxifen administration, when all genotypes were histologically comparable and similar in proliferation and apoptotic index. Disruption of RelA/p65 resulted in a reduced severity of the hyperproliferation (Fig. 9 B-E), ergo mice exhibited a more differentiated phenotype as indicated by an increased villus-to-crypt cell ratio and alkaline phosphatase staining labeling absorptive enterocytes. (Fig. 9 F, G). The more differentiated phenotype was also confirmed by a higher expression of differentiation cell markers Muc-2, synaptophysin and sucrose-isomaltase marking goblet cells, enteroendocrine cells and absorptive enterocytes, respectively (Fig. 9 H). A comparative gene expression analysis on mRNA extracts of IEC comparing Rela$^{\Delta IEC}$, β-cat$^{c.a.}$ and β-cat$^{c.a.}$/Rela$^{\Delta IEC}$ mice 15 days after tamoxifen administration, revealed a marked downregulation of a large set of Wnt-targets in IEC of β-cat$^{c.a}$/Rela$^{\Delta IEC}$ mice. Performing a gene set enrichment analysis (GSEA) verified significant enrichment of the stem cell transcriptome gene set (van der Flier, van Gijn et al. 2009) in β-cat$^{c.a}$ mice, however upon additional depletion of RelA this effect was abrogated and a significant regulation of stem cell markers was not detectable any more in β-cat$^{c.a}$ mice (normalized enrichment score 2.58, p< 0.001; Fig. 9 I), conferring NF-κB a crucial role on the regulation of the stem cell transcriptome and therefore an influence on the development of adenoma formation caused by aberrant Wnt signaling. In a real-time PCR experiment upregulation of stem cell markers Lgr5, Ascl2, Tnfrsf19, Fstl1, Ephb3, Cd44, Rnf43, Igfbp4, Zfp503 and Sox9 could be verified in IEC of β-cat$^{c.a}$ mice (Fig. 10 A).

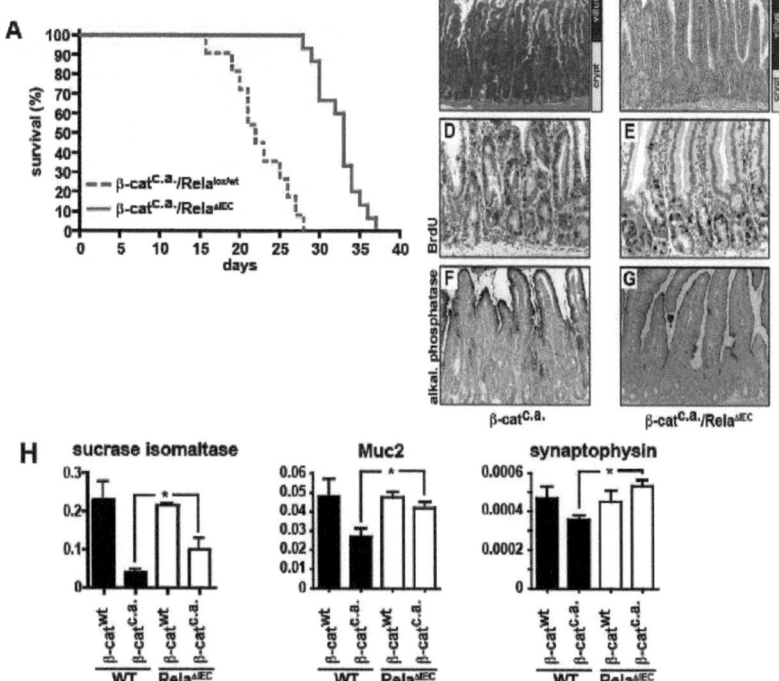

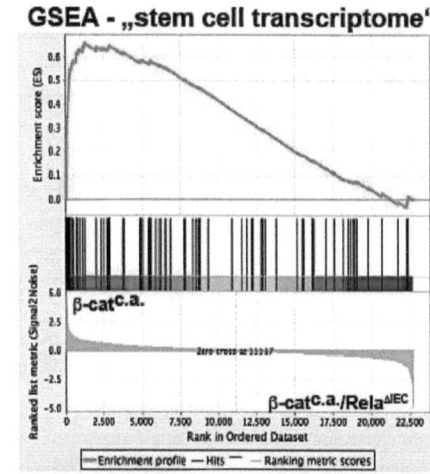

Normalized Enrichment Score (NES): 2.58
Nominal p-value: < 0.001

Figure 9: Loss of Rela in β-cat$^{c.a.}$ IEC prolongs survival and inhibits stem cell expansion

A colored version is available in the electronic edition

(A) Kaplan-Meier survival curve of β-cat$^{c.a.}$/Rela$^{lox/wt}$ (n=12) and β-cat$^{c.a.}$/Rela$^{\Delta IEC}$ mice (n=13), p= 0.0001 by log rank test. (B,C) H&E staining of β-cat$^{c.a.}$ and β-cat$^{c.a.}$/Rela$^{\Delta IEC}$ mice showing a higher villus/crypt ratio and less proliferation by (D,E) BrdU staining in β-cat$^{c.a.}$/Rela$^{\Delta IEC}$ mice (proliferation index: 0.31 ± 0.016 in β-cat$^{c.a.}$ mice versus

0.13 ± 0.006 in β-cat$^{c.a.}$/Rela^{ΔIEC} mice; n=3 of each genotype; p<0.0001). (F, G) Alkaline phosphatase staining of β-cat$^{c.a.}$ and β-cat$^{c.a.}$/Rela^{ΔIEC} mice. (H) RT-PCR expression analysis of duodenum IEC for differentiation markers sucrase-isomaltase, Muc2 and synaptophysin of wt, β-cat$^{c.a.}$, Rela^{ΔIEC} and β-cat$^{c.a.}$/Rela^{ΔIEC} mice on day 15. Data are mean ± SE; n≥3; analyzed using one-way ANOVA followed by Bonferroni post hoc test for multiple comparisons; only biologically relevant differences between genotypes are indicated; * p<0.05 (I) GSEA analysis comparing transcriptomes of β-cat$^{c.a.}$ and β-cat$^{c.a.}$/Rela^{ΔIEC} demonstrates enrichment of stem cell markers in β-cat$^{c.a.}$ IEC.

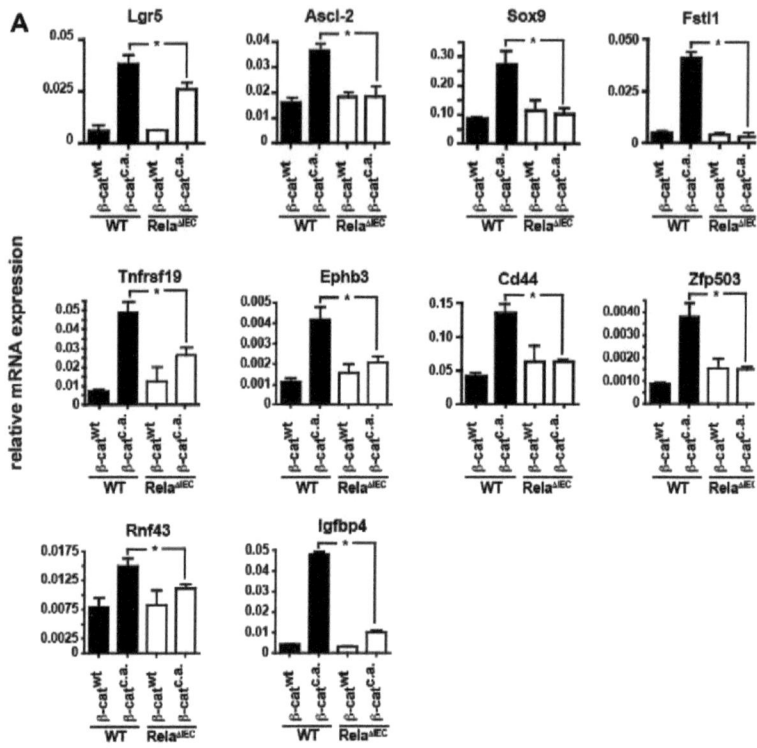

Figure 10: Loss of Rela in β -cat$^{c.a.}$ IEC is associated with decreased stem cell marker expression

(A) Relative mRNA expression analyzed by RT-PCR of intestinal stem cell markers in IEC of WT, β-cat$^{c.a.}$ Rela^{ΔIEC} and β-cat$^{c.a.}$/Rela^{ΔIEC} mice on day 15 of the model analyzed by Real-Time PCR. Data are mean ± SE; n≥3; analyzed using one-way ANOVA followed by Bonferroni post hoc test for multiple comparisons; only biologically relevant differences between genotypes are indicated; * p<0.05.

In order to study the molecular mechanism causing differential regulation of Wnt target genes in RelaA/p65 deficient β-cat$^{c.a.}$ mice, direct interference of NF-κB with β-catenin signal transduction was studied in primary IEC. As observed *in vitro* in various human cancer cell lines NF-κB and β-catenin are able to interact physically (Deng, Miller et al. 2002) and indeed interaction between both key factors can be detected *in vivo* in wildtype animals by performing immunoprecipitation from primary IEC, which is enhanced upon mutational stabilization of β-catenin in β-cat$^{c.a.}$ mice. (Fig. 11 A). A DNA affinity precipitation assay (DAPA) using a biotinylated Tcf/Lef consensus sequence confirmed enhanced binding capacity of stabilized β-catenin to DNA while binding was reduced in the absence of RelA/p65 (Fig. 11 B). Chromatin-immunoprecipitation (ChIP) verified the interaction of RelA/p65 with β-catenin on the promoter sequences of Wnt-targeted stem cell genes. A sequential ChIP (Re-ChIP) gave further prove for the simultaneous presence of both transcription factors at the same promoter regions (Fig. 12 A, B).

An *in vitro* approach using Hek 293 cells transfected with a constitutively active S33Y mutant of β-catenin along with wildtype Tcf4 confirmed that the observed changes in the DNA-binding are indeed part of cell internal regulations independent of variable amounts of different cell types due to changes in the villus/crypt ratio in the mouse intestine of different genotypes. Stimulation with TNF-α showed enhanced binding capacity of β-catenin to TCF/LEF consensus sequence in a DAPA experiment (Fig. 12 C). Various transfected amounts of a constitutively active form of IKKβ (IKKβ^{EE}) (Delhase, Hayakawa et al. 1999) revealed a dose-dependent binding activity of β-catenin and interaction of β-catenin and RelA/p65 with Tcf4 as well as CBP, which is known to be a common co-activator of NF-κB and of β-catenin (Fig. 12 D) (Najdi, Holcombe et al. 2011; Archbold, Yang et al. 2012). Conversely, knockdown of CBP via siRNA prevented the TNF-α-dependent increase in Wnt-reporter activity (Fig. 12 E) and abolished the interaction of RelA/p65 with β-catenin (Fig. 12 F) indicating that NF-κB mediated recruitment of CBP is crucial for its interaction with β-catenin in order to modify Wnt target gene transcription.

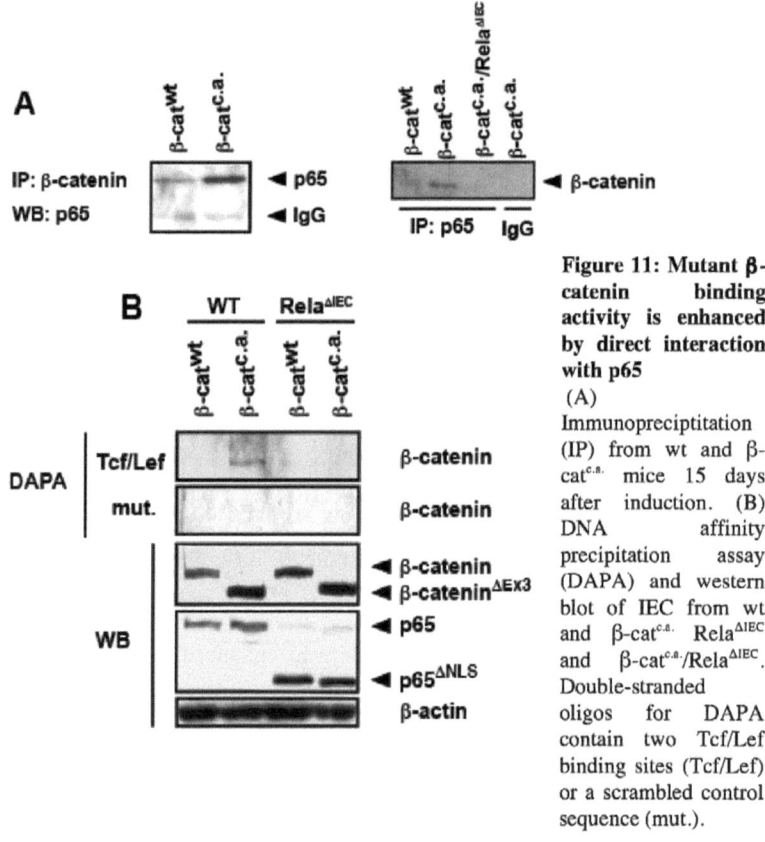

Figure 11: Mutant β-catenin binding activity is enhanced by direct interaction with p65
(A) Immunopreciptitation (IP) from wt and β-cat$^{c.a.}$ mice 15 days after induction. (B) DNA affinity precipitation assay (DAPA) and western blot of IEC from wt and β-cat$^{c.a.}$ Rela^{ΔIEC} and β-cat$^{c.a.}$/Rela^{ΔIEC}. Double-stranded oligos for DAPA contain two Tcf/Lef binding sites (Tcf/Lef) or a scrambled control sequence (mut.).

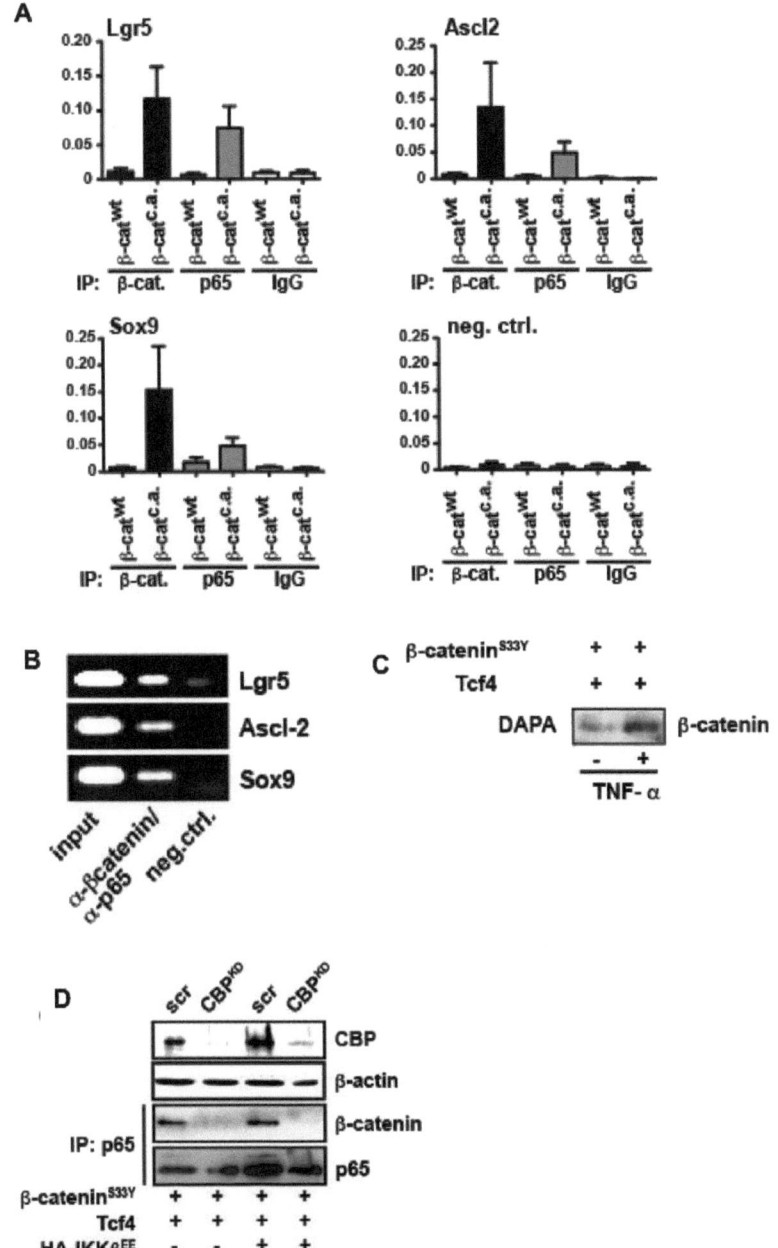

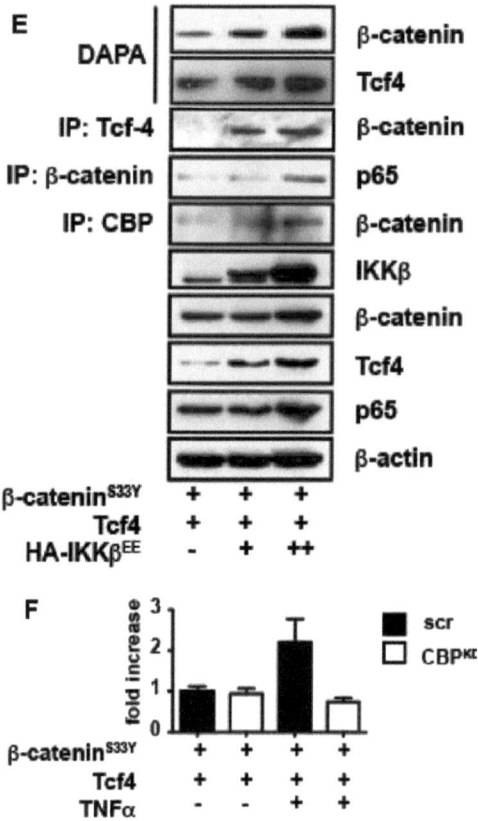

Figure 12: Dose dependent binding of β-catenin to intestinal stem cell promoter sequences by binding of p65 depending on the common co-activator CBP *in vivo* and *in vitro*

(A) Chromatin immunoprecipitation (ChIP) for β-catenin, p65 or EGFR as a negative control on DNA isolated from IEC of wt and β-cat[c.a] mice 15 days after tamoxifen administration. Precipitated DNA or 10% of chromatin input was amplified using promoter specific primers for Lgr5, Ascl-2, Sox9, which contain β-catenin/Tcf consensus motifs (Yochum, McWeeney et al. 2007) but no classical NF-κB-binding sites or a non-promoter region of EF1α (negative control). Data are mean ± SE; n≥4 (B) Re-ChIP assay on DNA isolated from IEC of a β-cat[c.a] mouse 15 days after tamoxifen administration using a β-catenin antibody for the first precipitation and p65 antibody for the second immunoprecipitation (except negative control) (C) DAPA for β-catenin from Hek 293 cells transfected with β-catenin[S33Y] and Tcf-4 and stimulated for 1h with 10 ng/mL TNF-α. (D) DAPA, IP and WB from Hek 293 cells transfected with β-catenin[S33Y], Tcf-4 and either 0, 0.5 or of 1 mg of a constitutively active form of IKKβ (IKKβ[EE]) (E) WB from lysates of Hek 293 cells transfected with β-catenin[S33Y] and Tcf-4 as well as either a siRNA pool for knockdown of CBP or scrambled siRNA pool as a negative control. (F) Luciferase assay on lysates from untreated or TNF-α stimulated (8h, 10 ng/mL) Hek 293 cells transfected with β-catenin^{S33Y}, Tcf-4, a Tcf/Lef reporter (TOPflash) sequence and scramble siRNA or a CBP targeting siRNA pool.

3.1.3 Enhanced NF-κB activity accelerates aberrant Wnt signaling-dependent crypt stem cell hyperproliferation and induces de-differentiation in non-stem cells

In order to find out whether enhanced NF-κB activity was able to aggravate the β-cat$^{c.a.}$-dependent phenotype of crypt cell hyperproliferation, β-cat$^{c.a.}$ mice were bred with floxed Iκbα mice (Rupec, Jundt et al. 2005) leading to a constitutively active NF-κB pathway in addition to constitutively active Wnt-signaling in β-cat$^{c.a.}$/Iκba^{ΔIEC} mice. Expectedly, loss of Iκba resulted in strengthened NF-κB activity and enhanced the development of crypt compartment expansion as the mice succumbed their phenotype already after a median survival of 15 days, a 32% shorter survival rate than β-cat$^{c.a.}$ mice (Fig 13 A, B). In line with elevated NF-κB activity, enhanced β-catenin activity was observed due to enhanced recruitment of CBP via NF-κB (Fig. 13 C). In addition to a massive hyperproliferation of the crypts, β-cat$^{c.a.}$/Iκba^{ΔIEC} double mutants frequently displayed aberrant crypt like foci along the villous epithelium (Fig. 14 A), which were highly proliferative including nuclear accumulation of β-catenin and showed expression of the stem cell marker c-myc (Fig. 14 B, C, D). Moreover, crypt-resembling foci expressed EphB3 (Fig. 14 F), which was formerly described to prevent directed migration of crypt cells to the tip of the villi in APC deficient epithelial cells and instead reside in the crypt compartment and fuel hyperproliferation (Battle 2002). Analogously, EphB3 expressing aberrant crypt foci detached from the surrounding villous epithelium and invaded into the subepithelium where they formed adenomatous crypts (Fig. 14 K). Furthermore, the expression of stem cell markers such as Ascl-2 or Sox-9 and most importantly, a strong positive in situ hybridization signal for the multipotent stem cell marker Lgr5 and Rnf43 in aberrant crypt foci lead to the assumption that aberrant crypt foci arose de novo in the villous epithelium due to acquisition of stem cell characteristics where they start adenomatous proliferation from the top down. These findings are in contrast to the bottom-up hypothesis, which has been proven recently by Barker et al. (Barker, Ridgway et al. 2009) claiming that Lgr5- positive multipotent crypt stem cells are the cells of origin of intestinal cancer. However, the described findings suggest NF-κB, as a strong modulator of the Wnt-dependent stem cell transcriptome, to initiate a de-differentiation program and re-expression of stem cell markers in aberrant location, the differentiated villous cells, where they can give rise to adenomatous crypts (Fig. 14 G-J).

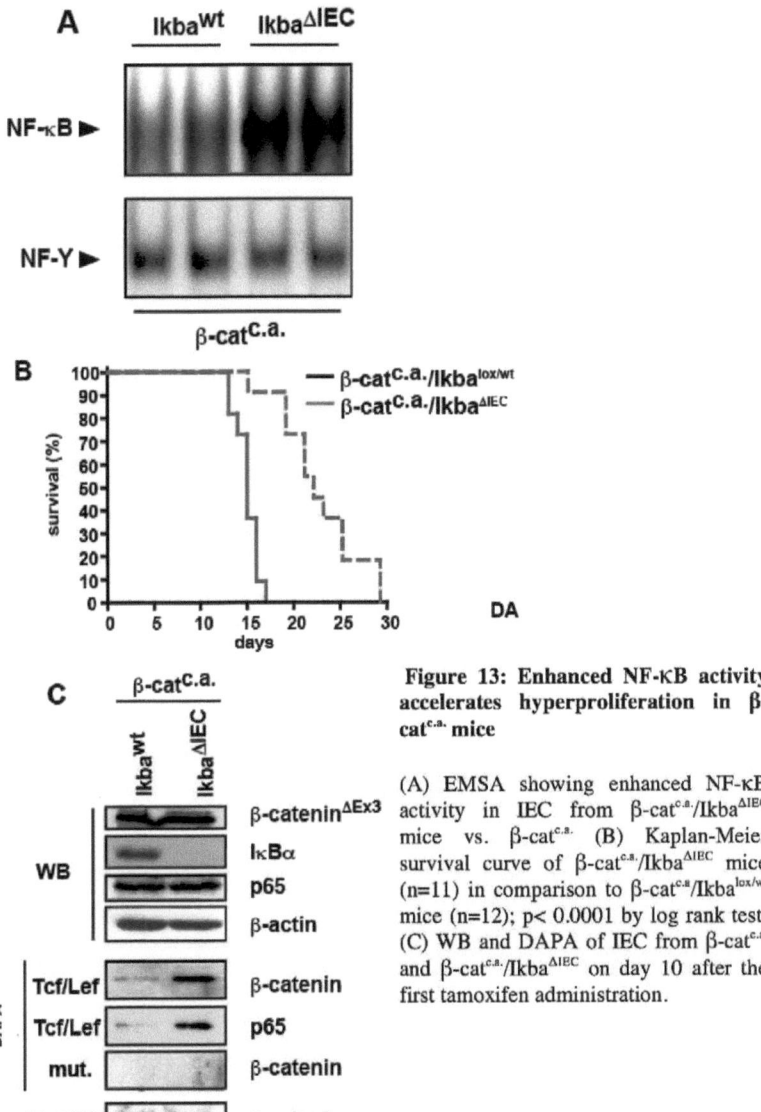

Figure 13: Enhanced NF-κB activity accelerates hyperproliferation in β-cat$^{c.a.}$ mice

(A) EMSA showing enhanced NF-κB activity in IEC from β-cat$^{c.a.}$/Ikba^{ΔIEC} mice vs. β-cat$^{c.a.}$. (B) Kaplan-Meier survival curve of β-cat$^{c.a.}$/Ikba^{ΔIEC} mice (n=11) in comparison to β-cat$^{c.a.}$/Ikba$^{lox/wt}$ mice (n=12); p< 0.0001 by log rank test. (C) WB and DAPA of IEC from β-cat$^{c.a.}$ and β-cat$^{c.a.}$/Ikba^{ΔIEC} on day 10 after the first tamoxifen administration.

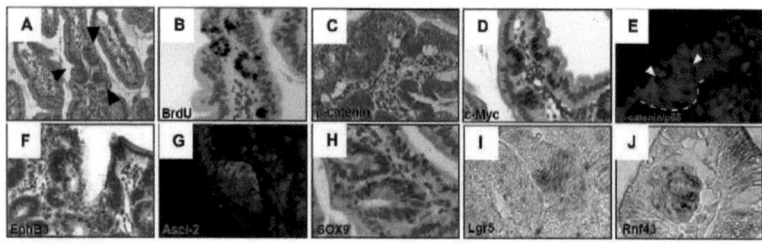

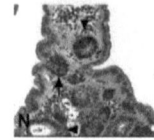

Figure 14: Enhanced NF-κB activity accelerates hyperproliferation and induces dedifferentiation of villous cells in β-cat$^{c.a.}$ mice

A colored version is available in the electronic edition

(A) H&E staining of β-cat$^{c.a.}$/Ikba^{ΔIEC} duodenum indicating aberrant crypt like foci in the villous compartment on day 10 after first tamoxifen administration. Immunohistochemical analysis reveals proliferation of aberrant crypt foci by (B) BrdU, (C) nuclear β-catenin and (D) c-myc expression in β-cat$^{c.a.}$/Ikba^{ΔIEC} (E) Duolink proximity ligation assay visualizes direct endogenous protein interation (fluorescent signal) of β-catenin and RelA/p65 in β-cat$^{c.a.}$/Ikba^{ΔIEC} villous crypt like structures (dashed white line). Aberrant villous crypts express stem cell markers (F) EphB3, (G) ASCL-2 and (H) SOX9. In situ hybridization revealed re-expression of stem cell markers (I) Lgr5 and (J) Rnf43 in aberrant villous crypts of β-cat$^{c.a.}$/Ikba^{ΔIEC}. (K) Immunohistochemical staining for c-myc expressed in villous subepithelial aberrant crypt foci (indicated by arrows) of β-cat$^{c.a.}$/Ikba^{ΔIEC} mice

3.1.4 Ex vivo dedifferentiated epithelial villus cells form spheroids with tumor stem cell capability

An established organoid culture system (Sato, Vries et al. 2009) served as a reliable method to test whether differentiated villus epithelial cells were indeed able to dedifferentiate and give rise to adenomatous crypt structures. Mechanically separated crypts and villi from villin-creER^{T2}/Apc$^{lox/lox}$ (termed Apc^{ΔIEC} hereafter) or villin-creER^{T2}/Apc$^{lox/lox}$/K-ras$^{G12D/+}$ mice (termed Apc^{ΔIEC}/K-ras^{G12D} hereafter) mice were used for growth in culture. Oncogenic K-Ras is known to enforce aberrant Wnt signaling (Bennecke et al., 2010; Janssen et al., 2006; Sansom et al., 2006) and to induce NF-κB activation (Perkins 2012) as was confirmed as well in crypt cells of $Apc^{\Delta IEC}$/K-ras^{G12D} animals, which displayed elevated NF-κB activity compared to crypts from $APC^{\Delta IEC}$ (Fig. 15 C). R-spondins are known enhancers of low-dose Wnt signals (Kazanskaya, Glinka et al. 2004). *in vivo*, R-spondin 1 strongly stimulates crypt proliferation (Kim, Kakitani et al. 2005). 2 days isolated after a single tamoxifen application wildtype crypts still were additionally dependent on Wnt signaling enhancer R-spondin for growth in culture, whereas cultured crypts derived from $Apc^{\Delta IEC}$ as well as $Apc^{\Delta IEC}$/K-ras^{G12D} formed adenomatous spheroids independent of extra R-spondin due to constitutively active Wnt signaling supported by oncogenic K-Ras and NF-κB (Fig. 15 A, B). Villi from $APC^{\Delta IEC}$ mice were not able to survive in culture without its supporting crypt niche isolated 2 days after a single tamoxifen application, while villi isolated from $Apc^{\Delta IEC}$/K-ras^{G12D} formed spheroids even in the absence of Wnt- signaling amplifying R-Spondin indicating autarky of external growth stimuli due to crypt-like characteristics including the capability of creating an independent growth niche (Fig. 15 D). However, application of the specific IKKβ- inhibitor ML120B (Nagashima, Sasseville et al. 2006) inhibited growth of $Apc^{\Delta IEC}$/K-ras^{G12D} villus cells and reduced spheroid formation of $Apc^{\Delta IEC}$/K-ras^{G12D} crypts by more than 60% (Fig. 15 D, E) underscoring the dependence of dedifferentiation on promoting NF-κB activity. After several passages of spheroids originating from $Apc^{\Delta IEC}$/K-ras^{G12D} villi or crypts, spheroids were still morphologically similar (Fig. 15 F) and kept their shape and size (Fig. 15 J). Injection of both, villi or crypt derived, spheroid types into nude mice revealed tumor growth with comparable growth kinetics in both cases (Fig. 15 K). Importantly, histological characterization of the formed tumors from crypt and villus derived spheres demonstrated expression of the multipotent stem cell marker

Lgr5 in both tumors of differing origin (Fig. 16 A). The de novo generation of Lysozyme positive Paneth cells within tumors of either origin further underlines the autonomy and the stem cell potential of tumor cells re-expressing Lgr5 (Fig. 16 A). In order to test whether villus derived cells showed tumor stem cells capabilities, villus derived spheroid cells were sorted by Lgr5+ and Lgr5- expressing cells and injected into nude mice. Interestingly tumors were formed from either cell population with similar growth kinetics and tumors derived from initially Lgr5- expressing cells displayed re-expression of Lgr5+ (Fig. 16 B, C, D), confirming their cancer stem cell potential of cells resulting from a dedifferentiation event.

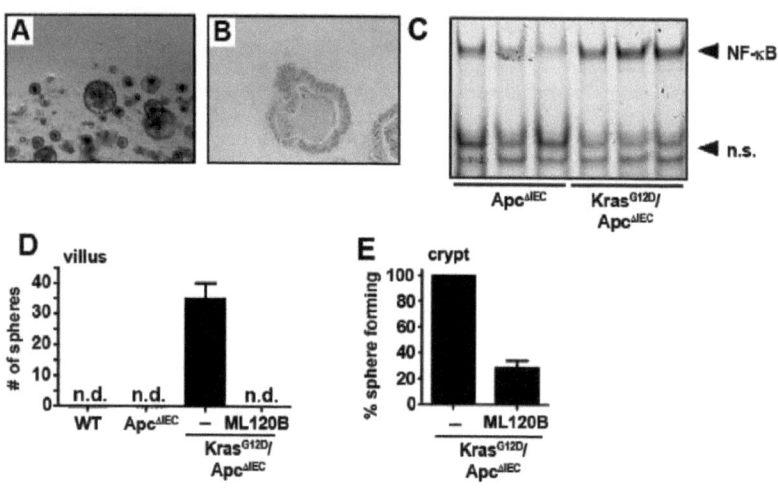

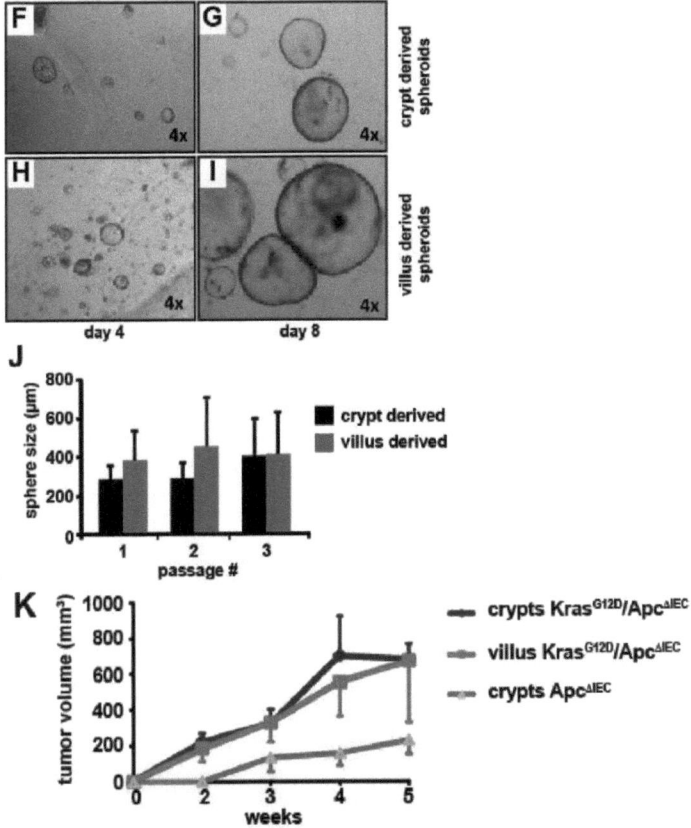

Figure 15: NF-κB dependent *ex vivo* dedifferentiation and cancer stem cell generation of Apc$^{\Delta IEC}$/K-ras^{G12D} derived villus cells

(A, B) Depiction of R-spondin independent spheroids generated of crypts from Apc$^{\Delta IEC}$ mice. (C) Increased NF-κB activity in crypts from Apc$^{\Delta IEC}$/K-ras^{G12D} compared to Apc$^{\Delta IEC}$ mice. (D, E) Quantification of formed spheroids derived from (D) villi and (E) crypts of Apc$^{\Delta IEC}$/K-ras^{G12D} and Apc$^{\Delta IEC}$ mice with and without IKKβ inhibitor ML120B treatment (n=5/genotype; n.d.: not detectable). (F-I) Depiction of crypt or villus-derived spheroid morphology from Apc$^{\Delta IEC}$/K-ras^{G12D} mice after (F, H) 4 and (G, I) 8 days in culture. (J) Sphere formation assay comparing crypt and villus-derived spheres derived from Apc$^{\Delta IEC}$/Kras^{G12D} mice. (K) Tumor growth in CD1 athymic mice after subcutaneous injection of crypt or villus-derived spheroids originating from Apc$^{\Delta IEC}$/K-ras^{G12D} and Apc$^{\Delta IEC}$ mice.

Data resulted from a collaboration with Owen Sansom and were produced by Patrizia Cammareri.

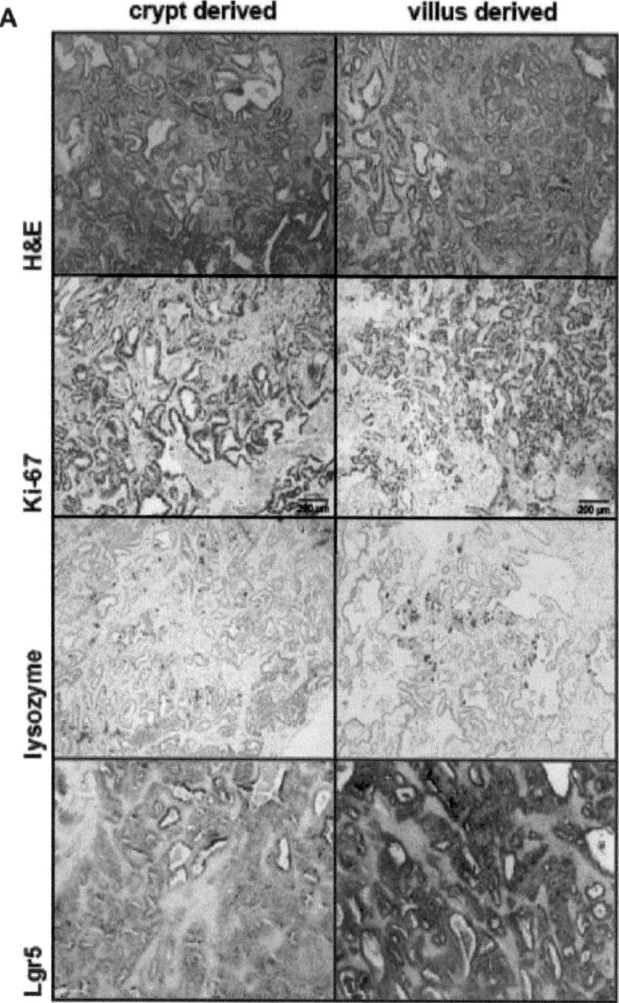

Figure 16: Tumor cells of Lgr5+ and Lgr5- spheroids either villus or crypt derived origin re-express stem cell marker Lgr5+ and display tumor stem cell characteristics

(A) Comparative histological analysis of tumors grown in CD1 athymic mice 22 days after the subcutaneous injection of crypt or villus derived spheroids originating from $Apc^{\Delta IBC}/K\text{-}ras^{G12D}$ mice. Lgr5 expression was detected by in situ hybridization

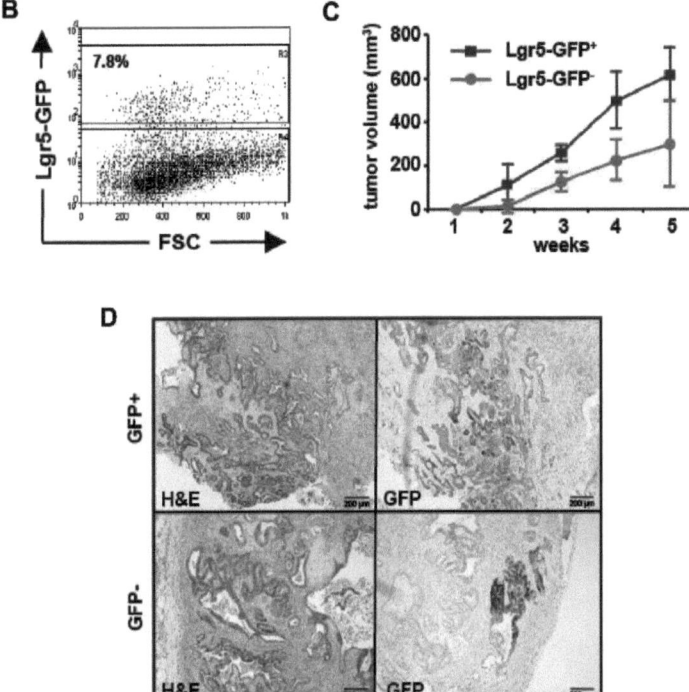

A colored version is available in the electronic edition

Figure 16: Tumor cells of Lgr5+ and Lgr5- spheroids either villus or crypt derived origin re-express stem cell marker Lgr5+ and display tumor stem cell characteristics

(B) FACS plot of villus derived spheroids from an Apc$^{\Delta IEC}$/K-ras^{G12D}/Lgr5-EGFP-IRES-creER^{T2} mouse sorted for Lgr5+ (GFP+ population). Absence of Lgr5 in the GFP- population was confirmed by PCR. (C) Growth characteristics of tumors resulting from subcutaneous injection of equal numbers of Lgr5+ or Lgr5- cells from villus-derived spheroids in CD1 athymic mice. (D) Immunohistochemistry of EGFP indicates expression of Lgr5 in tumors originating from Lgr5+ or Lgr5- villus cells.

Data resulted from a collaboration with Owen Sansom and were produced by Patrizia Cammareri.

3.1.5 Recombination in differentiated enterocytes leads to de-differentiation and adenoma formation *in vivo*

Since villin- Cre activity induces recombination in all intestinal epithelial cells including crypt cells, crypt-like foci in β-cat$^{c.a.}$/ IκBα$^{\Delta IEC}$ mice could have originated from the Lgr5+ stem cells at the base of the crypt and migrated upwards. To prove *in vivo* that adenomatous crypts evolved from non-stem cell villous epithelium, a mouse model was generated which allows Cre-recombination exclusively in Lgr5- differentiated enterocytes, but not in Lgr5+ multipotent crypt stem cells. According to Heijmans et al. a key mechanism associated with differentiation and cell homeostasis is endoplasmatic reticulum (ER)-stress and the subsequently induced unfolded protein response (UPR), whose activity was detected to be low in intestinal stem cells, while UPR occurred at high levels in transit amplifying (TA) cells and differentiated epithelial cells under normal homeostatic conditions (Heijmans et al, unpublished observations). A key component of the ER stress UPR response is the transcription factor X-box-binding protein 1 (XBP1) containing a bZIP domain. It was first identified by its ability to bind to the X-box, a conserved transcriptional element in the promoter of the human leukocyte antigen (HLA) DR alpha (Liou, Boothby et al. 1990). XBP-1u is ubiquitously expressed but under conditions of ER-stress, the XBP-1u mRNA is processed by Serine/Threonine endoribonuclease IRE1 in the nucleus. IRE1 catalyses the excision of a 26 nucleotide unconventional intron from XBP-1 mRNA, in a manner mechanistically similar to pre-tRNA splicing. Removal of this intron causes a frame shift in the XBP-1 coding sequence resulting in the translation of a 376 amino acid (54 kDa) XBP-1s active isoform rather than the 261 amino acid (33 kDa), XBP-1u inactive isoform (Yoshida 2007). The ER-stress activated indicator construct (ERAI) (Iwawaki, Akai et al. 2004) was genetically modified by replacing the venus sequence fused to XBP-1 sequence behind the 26 nt splice site by the sequence of an inducible Cre- recombinase in order to generate mice expressing an inducible Cre- recombinase only upon splicing and activation of XBP1 in differentiated epithelium (Fig. 12 A-C and unpublished observations by Heijmans and van den Brink). Cre induced recombination in differentiated IEC was confirmed by lineage tracing using Xbp1s-creER^{T2}-Rosa26R-dtTomato mice (Fig. 17 A-C). FACS sorting for separation of RFP+ and RFP- cells and a subsequent PCR revealed that stem cell markers Lgr5 and Bmi1 are not expressed in RFP+ cells. Immunofluorescence confirmed expression of RFP in differentiated villus cells and in Paneth cells after 24h of recombination induction, while no signal was detected after 33 days in accordance with the normal homeostatic turnover of differentiated IEC which approximates 5-7 days for villus cells and around 4 weeks for Paneth cells which have a longer turnover period and reside at the bottom of the crypt. The absence of adenomatous transformation and a hyperproliferative phenotype in Xbp1s-creER^{T2}/Ctnnb$^{loxEx3/wt}$ further suggested a recombination in non-stem cells, while Lgr5-EGFP-IRES-creER^{T2}/Ctnnb$^{loxEx3/wt}$ succumbed the adenomatous transformation within a median survival of 45 days (Fig. 18 E). However, by enhancing β-catenin activity through additional NF-κB or oncogenic K-Ras activation, which is known to promote Wnt signaling (Janssen, Alberici et al. 2006; Sansom, Meniel et al. 2006; Bennecke, Kriegl et al. 2010) and activate NF-κB (Fig. 15) (Perkins 2012), using homozygous Xbp1s-creER^{T2}/Ctnnb$^{loxEx3/loxEx3}$/Iκbα$^{lox/lox}$ mice or Xbp1s-creER^{T2}/Ctnnb^{loxEx3}/Kras^{G12D} initiation of adenomatous polyp formation led to death within 30 days (Fig. 19 A, C). The polyps were actively proliferating (Fig. 19 A) and re-expressed stem cell markers Rnf43 and Lgr5 as well as a number of genes belonging to the stem cell transcriptome, which gives genetic evidence for a de-differentiation process and extends the hitherto cell-of-origin hypothesis by differentiated Lgr5 negative cells as possible cells-of-origin (Fig. 19 D, E).

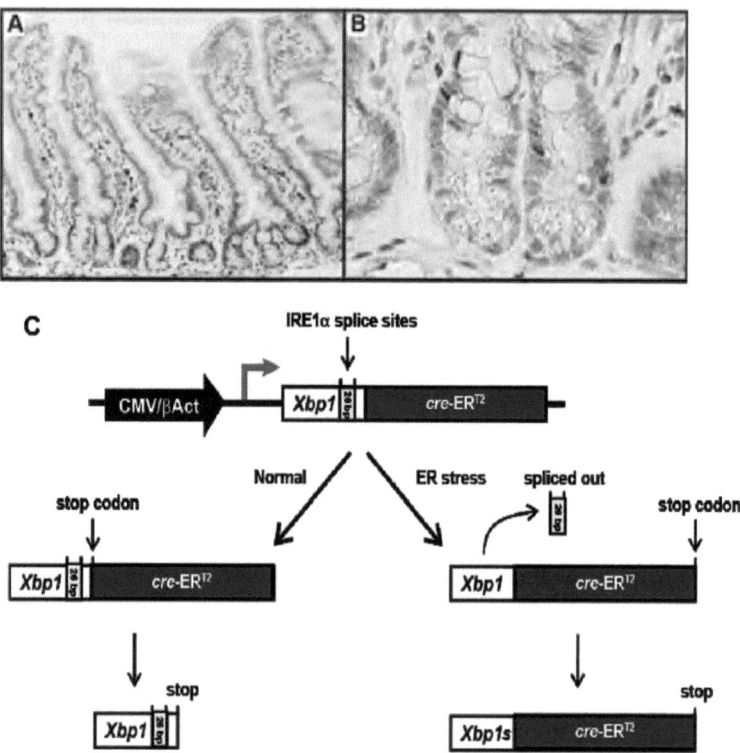

Figure 17: Generation of a mouse model allowing Cre-recombination exclusively in differentiated enterocytes, but not in Lgr5+ multipotent crypt stem cells

(A, B) Immunohistochemial staining of Xbp in wt mice demonstrating XBP expression only in Lgr5- IEC at the crypt villus junction, in the transit amplifying compartment and Paneth cells but not in Lgr5+ cells. (C) For generating mice expressing Cre in Lgr5- cells, the original 'ER stress–activated indicator' (ERAI) construct (Iwawaki, Akai et al. 2004) was used to replace the coding sequence of the YFP variant venus with a cre-ER^{T2} sequence, thus a fusion protein of XBP-1 and cre-

ERT2 would be expressed only in Lgr5- cells which splice Xbp.

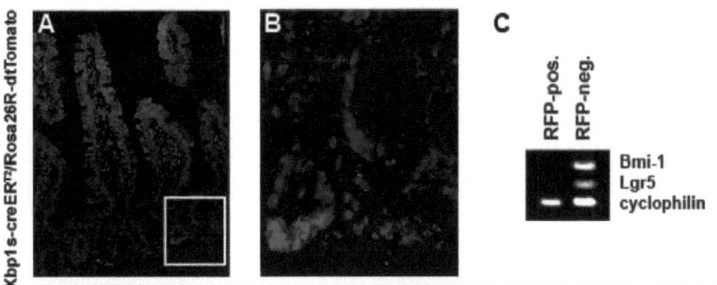

24h after 4-OHT

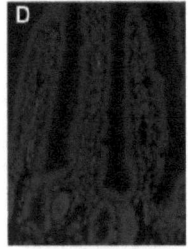

33d after 4-OHT

Figure 18: Xbp1s-creER^{T2} mice allow recombination only in non-stem cells

(A,B) RFP expression in Xbp1s-creER^{T2}-Rosa26R-tdTomato mice 24 hours after tamoxifen administration indicating recombination in (A) differentiated villous cells and in (B) Paneth cells. (C) PCR for Lgr5 and Bmi1 stem cells markers on cDNA of FACS sorted RFP+ and RFP- IEC confirming lack of stem cell marker expression in RFP+ cells of Xbp1s-creER^{T2} mice. (D) Lost RFP expression in IEC of Xbp1s-creER^{T2}-Rosa26R-tdTomato mice 33 days after tamoxifen administration.

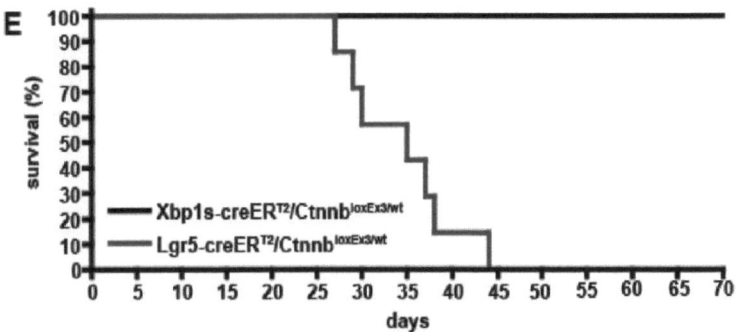

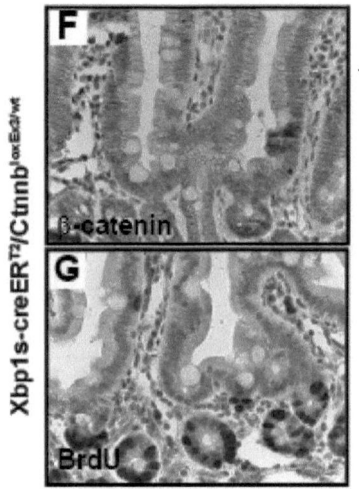

A colored version is available in the electronic edition

Figure 18: Xbp1s-creER^{T2} mice allow recombination only in non-stem cells

(E) Kaplan-Meier survival curve of Lgr5-IRES-EGFP-creER^{T2}/Ctnnb$^{loxEx3/wt}$ (n=7) and Xbp1s- creER^{T2}/Ctnnb $^{loxEx3/wt}$ (n=8) mice that were given the same amount of tamoxifen (5x1mg), p< 0.0001 by log rank test. Differences in survival between β-cat$^{c.a.}$ mice (Fig. 1A; villin-creER^{T2}/Ctnnb $^{loxEx3/wt}$) and Lgr5-IRES-EGFP creER^{T2}/Ctnnb$^{loxEx3/wt}$ mice is due to a lower recombination efficiency in Lgr5-IRES-EGFP-creER^{T2} mice causing a lower frequency of actual stem cell hits (Sansom et al., unpublished observation). Immunohistochemistry of (F) β-catenin and (G) BrdU in duodenum of Xbp1s-creER^{T2}/Ctnnb $^{loxEx3/wt}$ mice 50 days after the first tamoxifen administration displays sporadic positively stained cells outside the crypt compartment

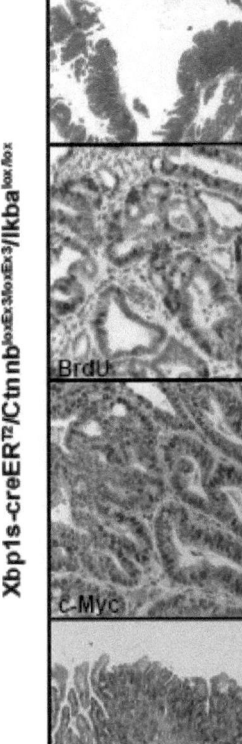

Figure 19: Dedifferentiation of non-stem cells allows initiation of tumorigenesis *in vivo*
(A) H&E staining and immunohistochemical analysis of BrdU incorporation and cmyc as well as in situ hybridization of Rnf43 in the proximal small intestine from a Xbp1s-creER^{T2}/Ctnnb$^{loxEx3/loxEx3}$/Iκbα$^{lox/lox}$ mouse 29 days after tamoxifen administration confirming re-expression of stem cell markers.

A colored version is available in the electronic edition

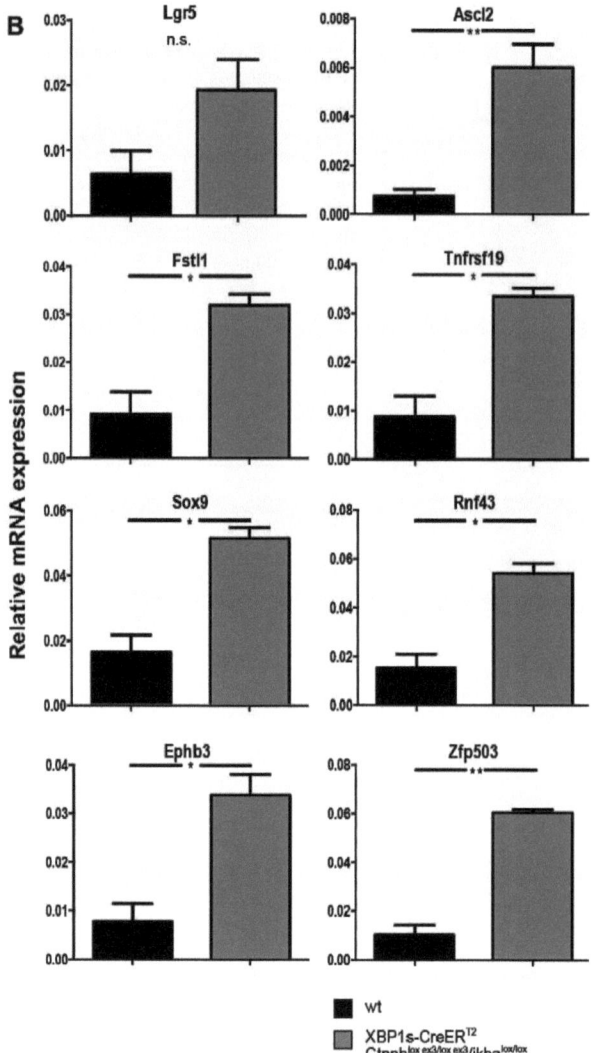

(B) Realtime-PCR of stem cell markers in IEC of wt and Xbp1s-creER^{T2}/Ctnnb$^{loxEx3/loxEx3}$/I$\kappa\beta^{lox/lox}$ mice 29 days after first tamoxifen application. Data are mean ± SE; n≥2; * p<0.05, analyzed by Student's t-test (Prism 6)

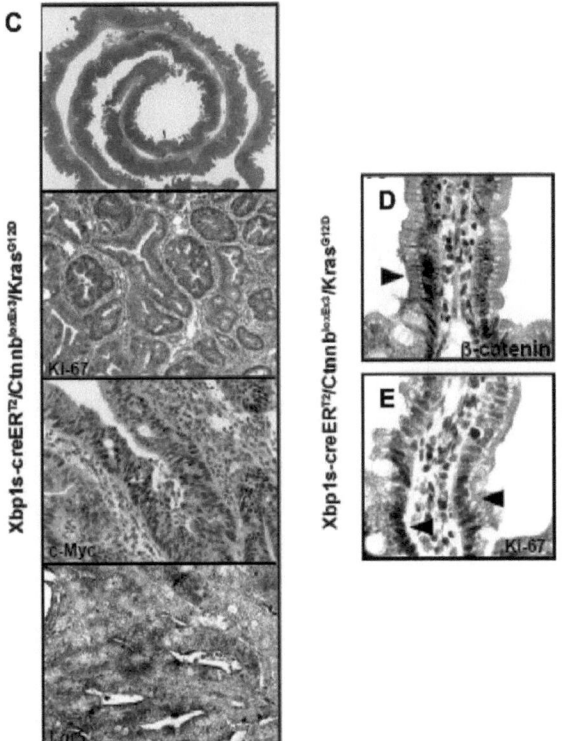

(C) H&E staining and immunohistochemistry of Ki-67 and c-myc as well as in situ hybridization confirming re-expression of Lgr5 in the proximal small intestine from a Xbp1s-creER^{T2}/Ctnnb^{loxEx3}/Kras^{G12D} mouse 29 days after tamoxifen administration. Immunohistochemical staining of (D) β-catenin and (E) Ki-67 in mice 24 hours after tamoxifen administration indicating recombination cells above the crypt-villus junction.

3.2 The role of NF-κB during tumor progression

3.2.1 Loss of p53 requires additional genetic mutation of Ctnnb in order to induce tumor formation and invasion

According to the genetic model of colorectal carcinogenesis accumulation of certain mutations in key tumor suppressor genes or oncogenes is necessary to enable the transition from a normal epithelial cell towards a metastasizing cancer cell (Fearon and Vogelstein 1990). While tumor initiation is usually induced by mutations in Wnt pathway components, tumor invasion and metastases formation are associated with the loss of the p53 tumor suppressive function in epithelial cells.

For investigating the role of p53 in the intestinal epithelium during Wnt dependent- tumor development, villin-Cre mice (Madison, Dunbar et al. 2002) were crossed to floxed Tp53 mice (Jonkers, Meuwissen et al. 2001) resulting in the deletion of exons 2-10 in the Tp53 gene in IEC (termed Tp53$^{\Delta IEC}$ hereafter). Under unchallenged circumstances the mice developed normally and were healthy and fertile. Intestinal architecture was preserved as differentiation, migration as well as cell proliferation and apoptosis were not affected (Fig. 20 A-H).

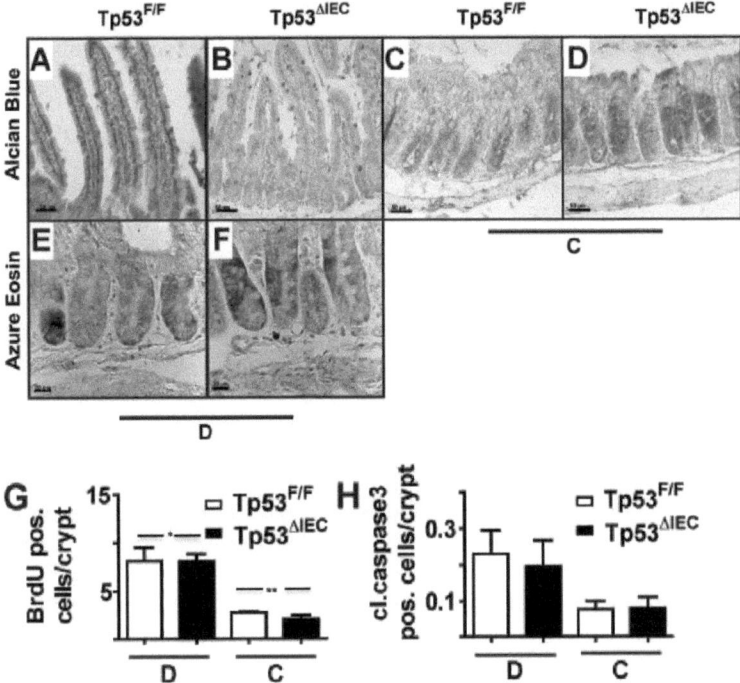

A colored version is available in the electronic edition

Figure 20: Histological characterization of unchallenged Tp53$^{\Delta IEC}$ revealed normal architecture comparable to littermate control mice

Alcian blue staining of (A,B) small intestine and (C,D) colon from unchallenged Tp53$^{\Delta IEC}$ and control mice depicting no noticeable difference in goblet cell appearance. (E,F) Azure Eosin staining of duodenum from unchallenged Tp53$^{\Delta IEC}$ and control mice showed normal Paneth cell occurrence. (G) BrdU index of proliferating crypt cells and (H) cleaved caspase 3 apoptotic index from immunohistochemically stained sections. Data are mean ± SE; n≥ 5 tumors of each genotype; analyzed by ANOVA followed by Bonferroni post hoc test for multiple comparisons, relevant comparison between Tp53$^{\Delta IEC}$ and control mice showed no significant differences. * p<0.05, ** p<0.001 for BrdU (G); cl. Casp 3 (H) exhibited no significant difference in any group.

During longterm observations for 14 months (n=20) unchallenged Tp53$^{\Delta IEC}$ mice did not show intestinal tumor development, suggesting that acquisition of additional mutations apart from p53 loss are necessary to lead to spontaneous formation of intestinal polyps. Since one of the first events during tumorigenesis in more than 80% of colonic tumors is ascribed to mutations in Wnt pathway components (Fodde, Smits et al. 2001), additional mutations in the Ctnnb gene were induced in Tp53$^{\Delta IEC}$ mice by repeated application of carcinogenic azoxymethane (AOM). AOM induces mutations in exon 3 of Ctnnb leading to accumulation of β-catenin and subsequent constitutive activation of the Wnt pathway (Greten, Eckmann et al. 2004). AOM challenged Tp53$^{\Delta IEC}$ mice displayed significantly increased tumor incidence in comparison to wildtype (wt) controls, while tumor size did not differ (Fig. 21 A, B), which was confirmed by a similar BrdU proliferation index and apoptotic index (Fig. 21 C, D) in both genotypes. Tumors of both genotypes were located in the colon, 18% of the Tp53$^{\Delta IEC}$ animals even developed tumors in the duodenum. Tumors from Tp53$^{\Delta IEC}$ mice grew highly invasive and after 16 weeks of tumor induction 50% of colonic tumors had invaded into the submucosa; after 20 weeks tumor invasion had even advanced through all intestinal tissue layers and had started extra-intestinal tumor growth (Fig. 22 E, F) while wt derived tumors never became invasive at any time point. Furthermore, local colonic lymph node metastasis could be detected in 30% of Tp53$^{\Delta IEC}$ mice (Fig. 22 G, H). Morphologically tumors from wt animals exhibited a tubular, more organized structure while tumor tissue from Tp53$^{\Delta IEC}$ mice was less differentiated (Fig. 22 C, D).

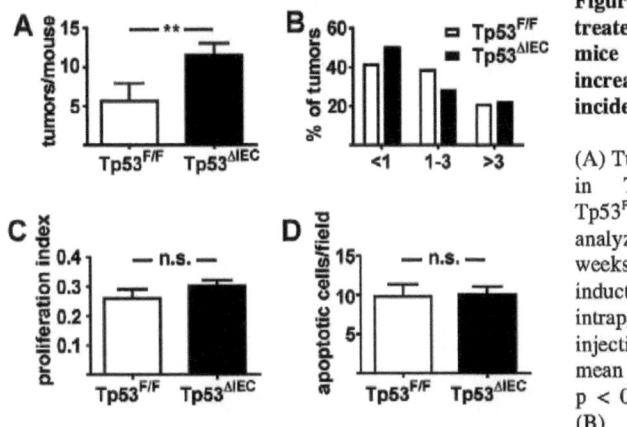

Figure 21: AOM treated Tp53$^{\Delta IEC}$ mice show increased tumor incidence

(A) Tumor incidence in Tp53$^{\Delta IEC}$ and Tp53$^{F/F}$ mice analyzed after 16 weeks after tumor induction by intraperitoneal AOM injections. Data are mean ± SE; n≥7; ** p < 0.001 by t-test. (B) Histogram showing size distribution of tumors. (C) BrdU proliferation index of epithelial tumor cells in AOM-induced tumors in Tp53$^{\Delta IEC}$ and Tp53$^{F/F}$ control mice. Data are mean ± SE; n≥10 tumors per genotype; n.s.: not significant, analyzed by two-tailed Student's t-test (D) Apoptotic index of tumor epithelial cells according to positive cleaved caspase 3 staining in AOM-induced Tp53$^{F/F}$ and Tp53$^{\Delta IEC}$ mice. Data are mean ± SE; n≥10 tumors of each genotype; n.s.: not significant, analyzed by two-tailed Student's t-test (Prism).

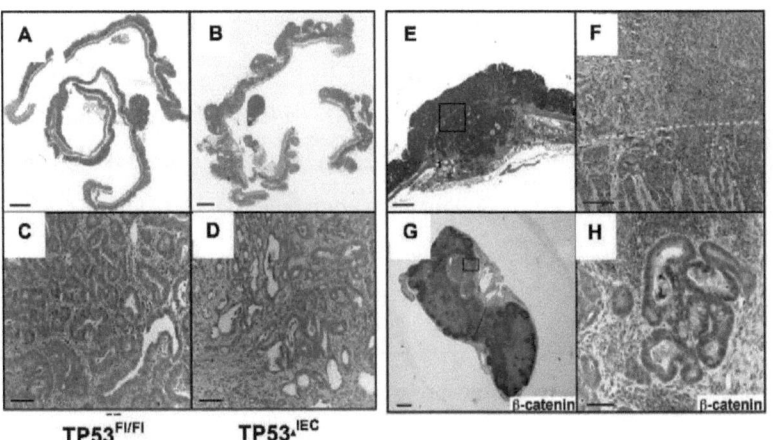

A colored version is available in the electronic edition

Figure 22: AOM treated Tp53$^{\Delta IEC}$ mice show aggressive invasion and metastases formation

(A-D) H&E staining of tumor bearing colon tissue from (A, C) control wt and (B, D) Tp53$^{\Delta IEC}$ mice 16 weeks after the first AOM-injection. Scale bars = 1000 μm (A, B) and 50 μm (C, D). (E, F) H&E staining of invasive colon carcinoma in AOM challenged Tp53$^{\Delta IEC}$ mice. Scale bars = 1000 μm (E) and 100 μm (F). (G, H) β-catenin immunohistochemical staining of a lymph node metastasis occurring in AOM-challenged Tp53$^{\Delta IEC}$ mice. Scale bars = 500 μm (G) and 50 μm (H).

3.2.2 p53 reduces the tumor incidence in Wnt- dependent tumorigenesis by inducing apoptosis and a DNA damage program in affected cells

In order to examine the cause of increased tumor incidence, AOM challenged Tp53$^{\Delta IEC}$ intestinal epithelium was tested for its initial apoptotic response to the carcinogen in comparison to Tp53$^{F/F}$ mice. In accordance with published results (Toft 1999; Greten 2004) in which it was known that AOM induced p53 dependent apoptosis within the first 8 hours of administration, this was not the case in p53-deficient animals, explaining the increased tumor incidence due to survival of AOM affected IECs (Fig. 23 A-C). This was associated with the decreased expression of pro-apoptotic proteins Bax, Puma, Noxa and Trail. Increased numbers of phospho- H2A.X IEC were correlating with decreased expression of Mgmt (Fig. 23 F), a protein mainly responsible for the repair of O^6-methylguanine containing DNA adducts (Fang, Kanugula et al. 2005) indicating DNA damaged cells (Fig. 23 D, E) which implicates an additional role for p53 in controlling DNA damage. To confirm the role of p53 in apoptosis of damaged cells as well as in induction of a DNA damage program, the effect of AOM on IEC was studied before and after p53 deletion using tamoxifen inducible villin-creER^{T2} mice (el Marjou, Janssen et al. 2004) and tumor incidence as well as extent of invasion in villin-creER^{T2}/Tp53$^{F/F}$ were compared. Expectedly, deletion of Tp53 preceding AOM administration led to a significantly higher tumor incidence (Fig. 24 B, C), but did not affect tumor size, suggesting that tumor incidence and tumor invasion are controlled independently by p53 (Fig. 24 D).

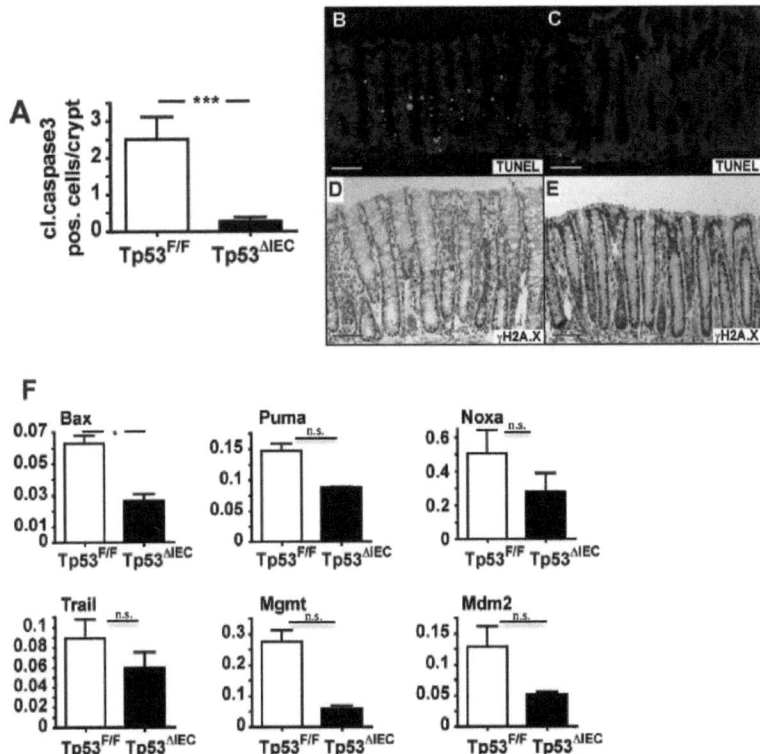

A colored version is available in the electronic edition

Figure 23: Impaired apoptotic induction and DNA damage response after deletion of p53

(A) Number of cleaved caspase 3 positive colonic IEC 8 hours after AOM injection in $Tp53^{F/F}$ and $Tp53^{\Delta IEC}$ mice. Data are mean ± SE of 50 crypts in two animals of each genotype; *** $p < 0.0001$ by t-test. (B, C) TUNEL staining (D, E) and immunohistochemical staining of DNA damage marker γH2A.X in colons sections of $Tp53^{\Delta IEC}$ and control $Tp53^{F/F}$ and mice 8 hours after AOM injection. Scale bars = 50 μm. (F) Relative mRNA expression levels of apoptosis related markers Bax, Puma, Noxa, Trail, Mgmt and Mdm2 in colonic IEC of $Tp53^{F/F}$ and $Tp53^{\Delta IEC}$ mice 8 hours after AOM injection. Data are mean ± SE; n≥2, * $p<0.05$ and n.s.= not significant, analyzed by Student's t-test (Prism 6).

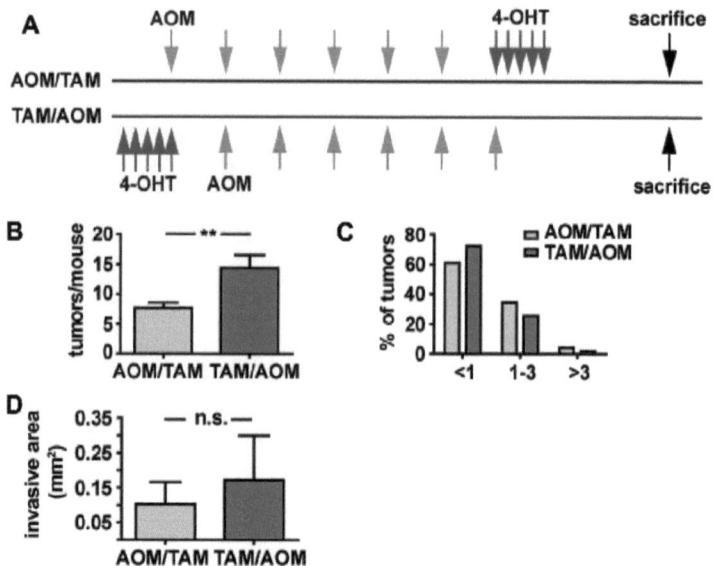

Figure 24: Tumor incidence and tumor invasion are controlled by p53 via different mechanisms
(A) Schematic overview depicting respective treatment approach for p53 deletion either before or after AOM application in tamoxifen inducible villin-creER^{T2}/Tp53$^{F/F}$ mice. (B) Tumor incidence in villin-creER^{T2}/Tp53$^{F/F}$ mice 16 weeks after tumor induction according to different time points of p53 deletion during the course of tumorigenesis as shown in (C). Data are mean ± SE; n ≥ 3; ** p < 0.001 by t-test (D) Histogram showing size distribution of tumors. (E) Average invasive area in colonic tumors of villin-creER^{T2}/Tp53$^{F/F}$ mice challenged with AOM before or after p53 deletion. Data are mean ± SE; n ≥ 3; n.s.: not significant.

3.2.3 Loss of Tp53 leads to a myeloid cell dominated inflammatory microenvironment associated with NF-κB activation facilitating EMT and invasion

Moreover, tumors of p53 deficient animals did not harbor any other considerable genomic instability as an array comparative genomic hybridization (CGH) analysis (data not shown) merely revealed a few insignificant chromosomal amplifications.

A microarray analysis of tumor tissue from Tp53$^{\Delta IEC}$ mice and littermate controls by using Affymetrix Mouse Genome 430A 2.0 Gene Chips revealed 370 significantly differentially regulated genes of which 223 were upregulated and 147 were downregulated by at least 2-fold in Tp53-deficient tumors compared to wildtype adenomas. According to functional classes upregulated genes could be categorized into genes associated with chemotaxis, prostaglandin synthesis and inflammation (Fig. 25 A), most notably Cxcl1, Cxcl2, Ptgs2 and IL-11, which could be verified by RT-PCR (Fig. 26 A). Furthermore, genes, associated with cell adhesion and morphogenesis, including Twist as a major regulator of epithelial-mesenchymal-transition (EMT), were upregulated (Kim et al., 2009; Polyak and Weinberg, 2009; Yang et al., 2004), conversely epithelial marker E-Cadherin was downregulated as a part of the EMT program (Fig. 26 B). Apart from that, matrix-modifying enzymes such as cathepsins and matrix metalloproteinases (Ctsl1, Mmp2, Mmp3, Mmp10 and Mmp13), crucial for the invasive process, were upregulated in Tp53-deficient tumors (Fig. 26 C).

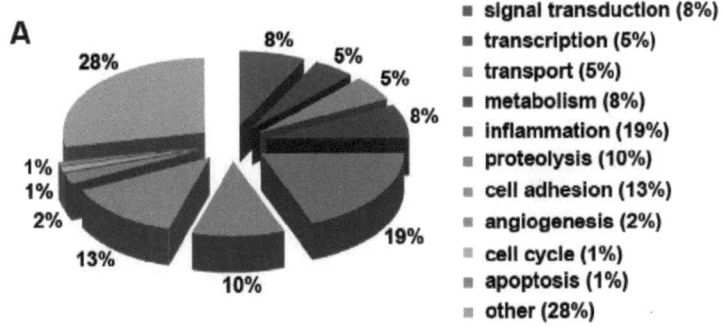

A colored version is available in the electronic edition

Figure 25: Percental proportion of functional gene classes upregulated in in Tp53$^{\Delta IEC}$ tumors

(A) Pie chart depiction of genes classified according to KEGG, which are more than 2-fold upregulated in invasive tumors from Tp53$^{\Delta IEC}$ mice compared to non-invasive adenomas from p53 proficient mice 16 weeks after the first AOM administration. The group "inflammation" contains genes involved in chemotaxis, inflammation and prostaglandin synthesis.

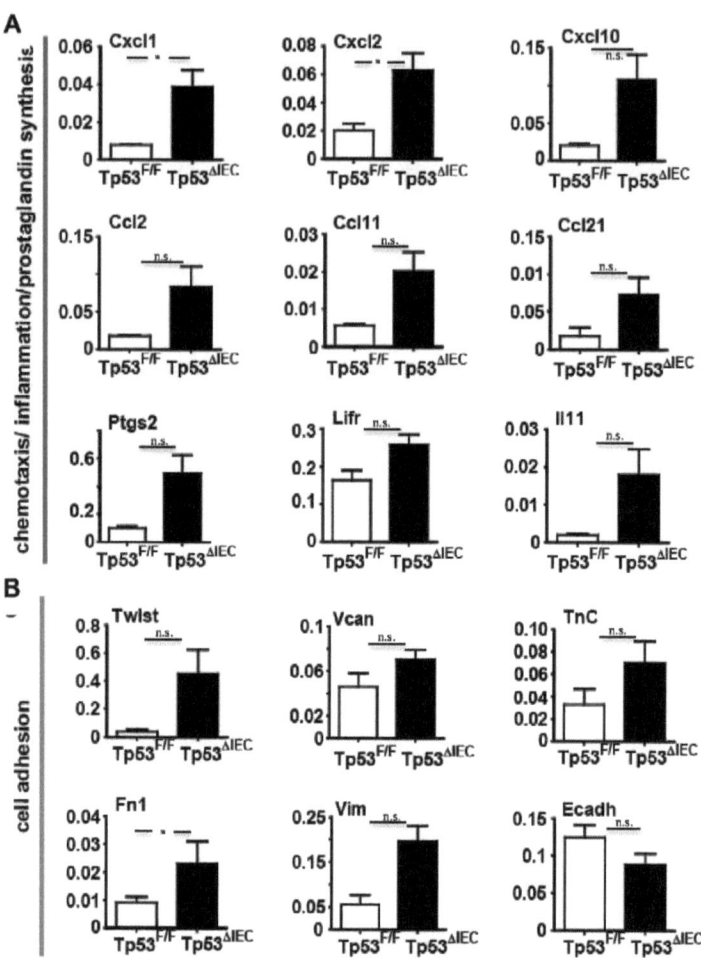

Figure 26: Upregulation of inflammatory and EMT markers in Tp53$^{\Delta IEC}$ tumors

(A-C) RT-PCR for relative mRNA expression levels of selected genes in tumors isolated from AOM-induced Tp53$^{F/F}$ and Tp53$^{\Delta IEC}$ mice. Data are mean ± SE; n ≥ 3, * p < 0.05 and n.s.= not significant, analyzed by two-tailed Student's t-test (Prism 6).

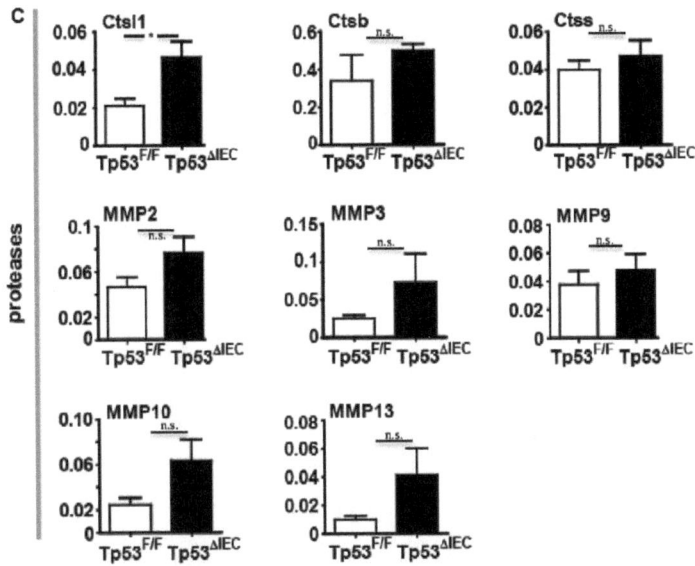

In human invasive colorectal cancer a particular set of NF-κB target genes is overexpressed specifically in cells of the invasive front compared to cells in the center of the same tumor (Horst, Budczies et al. 2009) including Cxcl1, Cxcl10, Ctsl1, Twist and Tenascin C. By comparing this NF-κB controlled invasion specific gene set with tumors from Tp53^{ΔIEC} mice in a cross-species gene set enrichment analysis (GSEA), indeed a significant correlation of this gene panel could be detected in p53 deficient tumors but not in wt tumor tissue (Fig. 27 A). In line, phosphorylation of Ikba and RelA/p65 as well as nuclear accumulation of phospho-p65 in tumor cells and stroma cells confirmed enhanced NF-κB activity (Fig. 27 B, C). Correlating with high expression of the powerful chemo-attractants Cxcl1, Cxcl2 and Ccl2 (Fig. 27 D) (Murdoch, Muthana et al. 2008), F4/80+ and Gr1+ myeloid cells were recruited to the basal membrane along the invasion front of tumors of Tp53^{ΔIEC} mice (Fig. 27 E, F), whereas immune cells were more evenly distributed in wt adenomas (Fig. 29 A-D). Western blots showing enhanced Twist expression in Tp53-deficient tumors and strong nuclear staining of mesenchymal markers Twist and Vimentin in invading tumor cells, which still expressed epithelial E-Cadherin, visualized the epithelial- mesenchymal transition process in p53-deficient tumors (Fig. 27 G, H, I).

In order to confirm a NF-κB dependent recruitment of an inflammatory microenvironment in human colorectal invasive cancers, a patient cohort consisting of 59 patients was analyzed for infiltration of neutrophils and macrophages as well as nuclear NF-κB activity and p53 nuclear accumulation indicating mutations of p53. Importantly, nuclear NF-κB staining and p53 mutations were found to correlate in surgically resected cancer specimens diagnosed with invasive colon cancer (Fig. 28 A-E). Moreover, activation of NF-κB correlated with the occurrence of lymph node metastases in this patient cohort (Fig. 28 F). Supportingly, enhanced recruitment of infiltrating CD68+ macrophages was correlating significantly with a p53 mutation/phospho-p65 positive status in the patient cohort (Fig. 28 G-I), however there was no significant enrichment of myeloperoxidase (MPO) positive neutrophils in any patient sample subgroup.

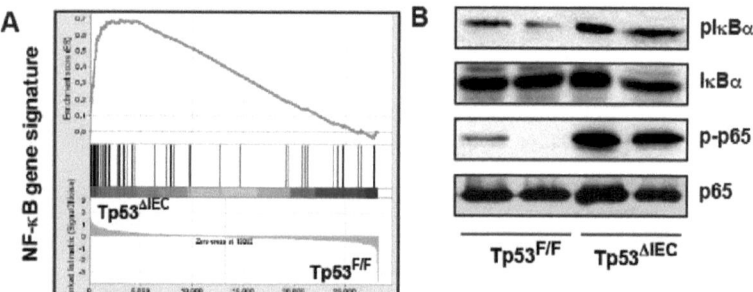

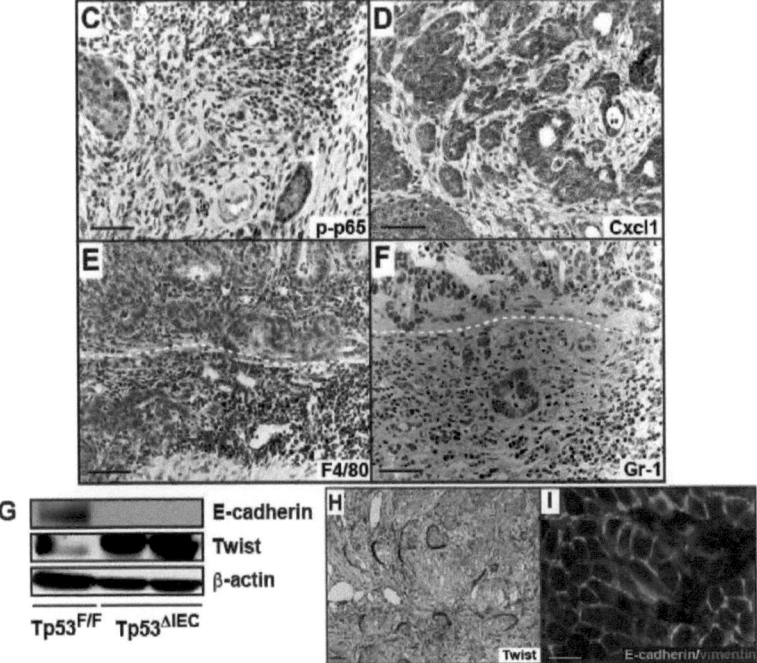

A colored version is available in the electronic edition

Figure 27: Enhanced NF-κB activation correlates with expression of EMT markers and recruitment of inflammatory cells in Tp53$^{\Delta IEC}$ mice

(A) Gene set enrichment analysis (GSEA) proving significant enrichment of a specific set of NF-κB target genes known to be upregulated at the invasive front of human invasive carcinomas (Horst, Budczies et al. 2009) in tumors from Tp53$^{\Delta IEC}$ mice. Normalized enrichment score (NES): 1.46; $p < 0.0001$. (B) Western blot analysis confirming NF-κB pathway activation in invasive colon tumor tissue from Tp53$^{\Delta IEC}$ mice 16 weeks after the first AOM administration. (C-F) Immunohistochemical staining of (C) p-p65, (D) Cxcl1, (E) F4/80 and (F) Gr-1 in and along invasive areas of AOM-challenged Tp53$^{\Delta IEC}$ colon tumors of mice. Dashed white line marks basal membrane. Scale bars = 50 μm. (G) Western blot showing inverse correlation of Twist and E-Cadherin expression in invasive cancers from Tp53$^{\Delta IEC}$ mice and non-invasive adenoma from control mice 16 weeks after the first AOM administration. (H) Immunohistochemistry of Twist in invasive tumors of AOM-challenged Tp53$^{\Delta IEC}$ (I) Co-localized epithelial E-cadherin and mesenchymal vimentin in invasive tumor areas indicate EMT in Tp53$^{\Delta IEC}$ mice; Nuclei are stained using DAPI (blue). Scale bar = 200μm. A colored version is available in the electronic edition.

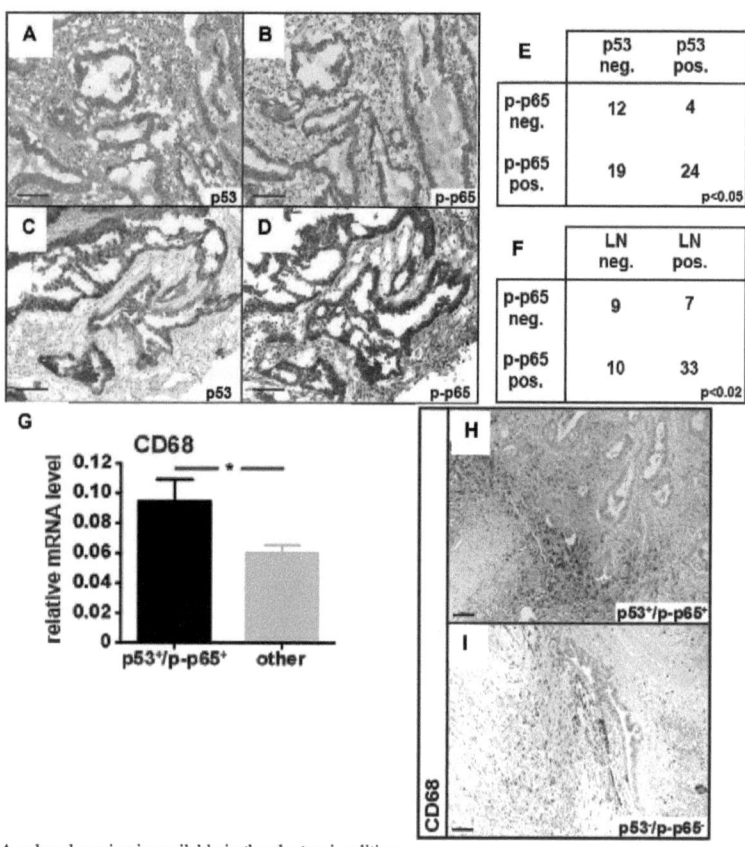

A colored version is available in the electronic edition

Figure 28: Correlation of p53 mutations and p65 nuclear localization with infiltration of CD68 macrophage infiltration and lymph node metastases occurrence in human colorectal cancer patients

(A-D) Immunohistochemical analysis of (A, C) mutant p53 (nuclear staining) and (B, D) activated p-p65 in human colorectal cancer tissue. Scale bars = 100μm. (E) Correlation of mutant p53 and p-p65 in human colorectal cancer patient cohort analyzed by Pearson's Chi-square test (n=59; χ2-test, p<0.05). (F) Correlation of p-p65 staining and presence of lymph node metastases according to Pearson's Chi-square test (n=59; χ2-test, p<0.02). (G) relative mRNA expression level of the macrophage specific marker CD68 correlating with positive phospho-p65 status in p53 mutation-bearing human colorectal tissue samples ("p53+/p-p65+"; n=23 and "other"; n=30). Data are mean ± SE; * p < 0.05 by t-test. Immunohistochemical staining of CD68 in (H) p53 mutated/phosphor-p65 positive samples comparing (I) p53 unmutated and phospho-p65 negative classified samples from human colon cancer patients. Scale bars = 100 µm.

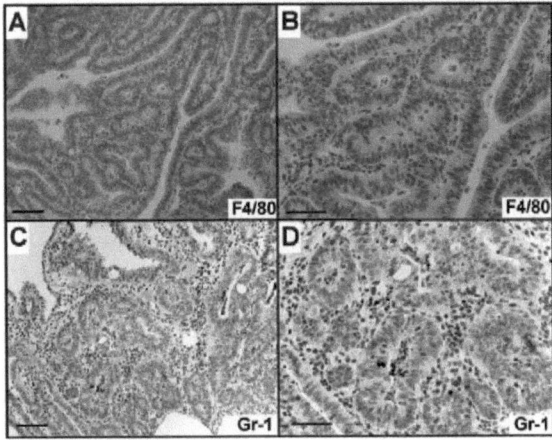

Figure 29: Immune cell infiltration in wt adenomas of Tp53$^{F/F}$ mice

Immunohistochemical analysis of (A,B) macrophage and (C,D) neutrophil infiltration in wt non-invasive adenomas. Scale bars = 50µm (B,C) and 100µm (A,C).

A colored version is available in the electronic edition

3.2.4 Loss of p53 leads to intestinal barrier defect after carcinogen exposition resulting in increased bacterial translocation and serum LPS levels activating NF-κB in IEC

To investigate whether a cell autonomous or non-autonomous mechanism was the cause of NF-κB activation, mice were injected with LPS in order to activate NF-κB in IEC (Egan, Eckmann et al. 2004). Formerly, it was shown in p53 deficient embryonic fibroblasts that increased interaction of p300/CBP and NF-κB or elevated levels of Glut3 were responsible for enhanced NF-κB activity intrinsically (Webster and Perkins 1999; Kawauchi, Araki et al. 2008), which however was not detectable in IEC of Tp53$^{\Delta IEC}$ mice (Fig. 30 A, B). In addition there was no enhanced expression of classic NF-κB target genes in p53-deficient IEC compared to p53 proficient control IEC proposing an external trigger for NF-κB activation in IEC of Tp53$^{\Delta IEC}$ mice.

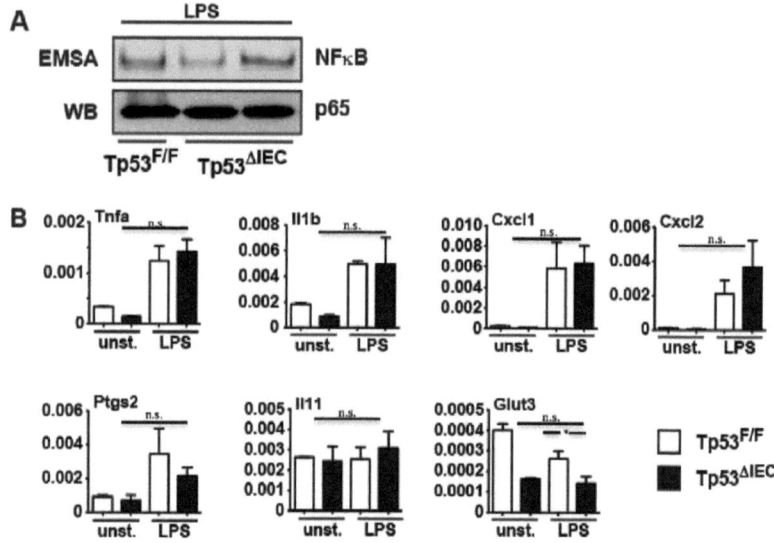

Figure 30: NF-κB activity does not differ between Tp53^{ΔIEC} and Tp53$^{F/F}$ mice after LPS treatment
(A) EMSA and RelA/p65 loading control blot for LPS induced NF-κB activity in colonic IEC comparing Tp53^{ΔIEC} and Tp53$^{F/F}$ mice. LPS was injected 1h before sacrifice. (B) relative mRNA expression levels of colonic IEC for depicted NF-κB target genes and Glut 3 showing no difference in fold-induction between Tp53^{ΔIEC} and littermate control mice 4h after LPS injection. Data are mean ± SE; n ≥ 3; analyzed by one-way ANOVA followed by Bonferroni post hoc test for multiple comparisons; * p < 0.05 and n.s.= not significant.

An impaired epithelial barrier and increased intestinal permeability can be found in human colon carcinomas and has been shown to be the case in carcinogen-induced colon carcinogenesis in rodents as well (Soler, Miller et al. 1999). This observation was confirmed by the fact that unchallenged Tp53^{ΔIEC} mice compared to control mice did not exhibit increased LPS plasma levels, whereas AOM challenged mice revealed a 2.5 fold elevated LPS plasma level in Tp53^{ΔIEC} mice in contrast to littermate controls (Fig. 31 A). Increased LPS levels seemed to result from enhanced attachment and infiltration of microfloral bacteria into

IEC and tumor IEC of Tp53$^{\Delta IEC}$ mice as fluorescence in situ hybridization (FISH) for the bacterial consensus sequence EUB338 revealed (Fig. 31 C, D). In line with altered tight junction permeability, expression of occludin, a major tight junction complex component, was decreased in IEC of Tp53$^{\Delta IEC}$ mice (Fig. 31 E, F). Apart from occludin expression levels, claudins, another class of important tight junction complex proteins, as well as JAM-A and Muc-1 expression were affected (Fig. 31 G). Elevated levels of claudin 1 and Muc-1 and decreased expression of claudin 2 and JAM-A have also been found in human colorectal cancer (Jang, Chae et al. 2002; Wang, Tully et al. 2011). Importantly, increased serum levels upon oral application of FITC-Dextran, an unpolarized high-molecular weight molecule, that is normally known to be prevented from intestinal nutrient uptake and passing intestinal barrier unless intestinal tight junction permeability is disrupted (Purandare, Offenbartl et al. 1989) (Fig. 31 B), measured one week after the last of repetitive AOM applications suggest that AOM administration attenuates protective intestinal barrier in Tp53$^{\Delta IEC}$ mice and leads to increased LPS plasma levels and NF-κB activation (Fig. 31 H; Fig. 32 A, B) long before invasive tumor growth. In order to conversely prevent NF-κB activation at this early time point, AOM challenged Tp53$^{\Delta IEC}$ mice were treated with an antibiotic cocktail consisting of vancomycin, metronidazole, ampicillin and neomycin for two weeks in the drinking water (Fig. 32 C). Depletion of intestinal microflora was confirmed by plating stool samples on blood agar plates. Indeed, treatment with antibiotics impaired NF-κB activation colon mucosa of AOM treated Tp53$^{\Delta IEC}$ mice (Fig. 32 D-F) consequently resulting in decreased expression of chemo-attractants Cxcl1, Cxcl2 and inflammation marker Ptgs2 (Fig. 32 G) confirming the impact of microfloral bacteria on initialization of NF-κB activity preceding tumor growth.

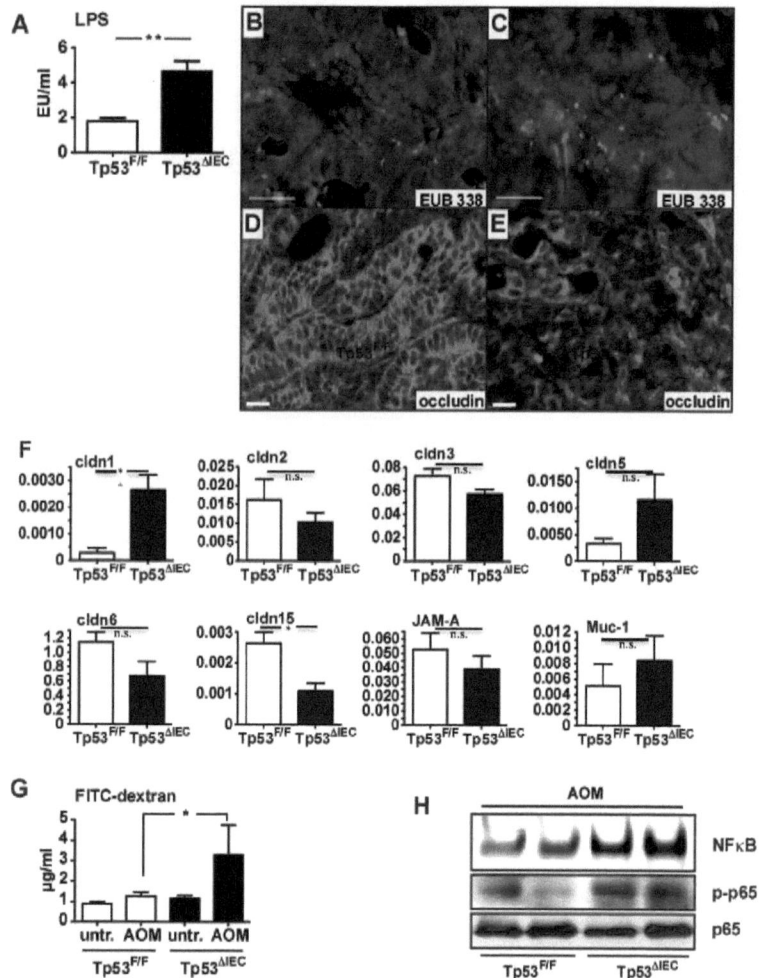

A colored version is available in the electronic edition

Figure 31: Tp53$^{\Delta IEC}$ mice develop an intestinal barrier defect upon carcinogen exposure

(A) LPS plasma levels analyzed from portal vein blood of Tp53$^{F/F}$ and Tp53$^{\Delta IEC}$ mice with AOM-induced tumors. Data are mean ± SE; n ≥ 3; ** p < 0.001 by t-test. (B, C) FISH using a FITC-labeled probe designed from a eubacterial consensus sequence (EUB 338) shows enhanced attachment and infiltration of intestinal bacteria into tissue of Tp53$^{\Delta IEC}$. (D, E) Immunofluorescence of occludin reveals decreased and irregular expression in (D) invasive tumor areas from Tp53$^{\Delta IEC}$ mice compared to (E) non-invasive adenomas in Tp53$^{F/F}$ mice. (F) Relative mRNA expression levels of selected intestinal barrier components in tumor tissues of Tp53$^{F/F}$ and Tp53$^{\Delta IEC}$. Data are mean ± SE; n ≥ 3, n.s.= not significant or * p < 0.05; analyzed by Student's t-test (G) FITC-dextran plasma levels analyzed 4 hours after oral gavaging in untreated Tp53$^{F/F}$ and Tp53$^{\Delta IEC}$ mice and one week after the last AOM-challenge preceding tumor growth. Data are mean ± SE; n =8; * p < 0.05 by one way ANOVA followed by post hoc Bonferroni for multiple comparisons. (H) EMSA and western blot analysis for NF-kB activation in colon tissue from Tp53$^{F/F}$ and Tp53$^{\Delta IEC}$ mice four weeks after the last AOM application.

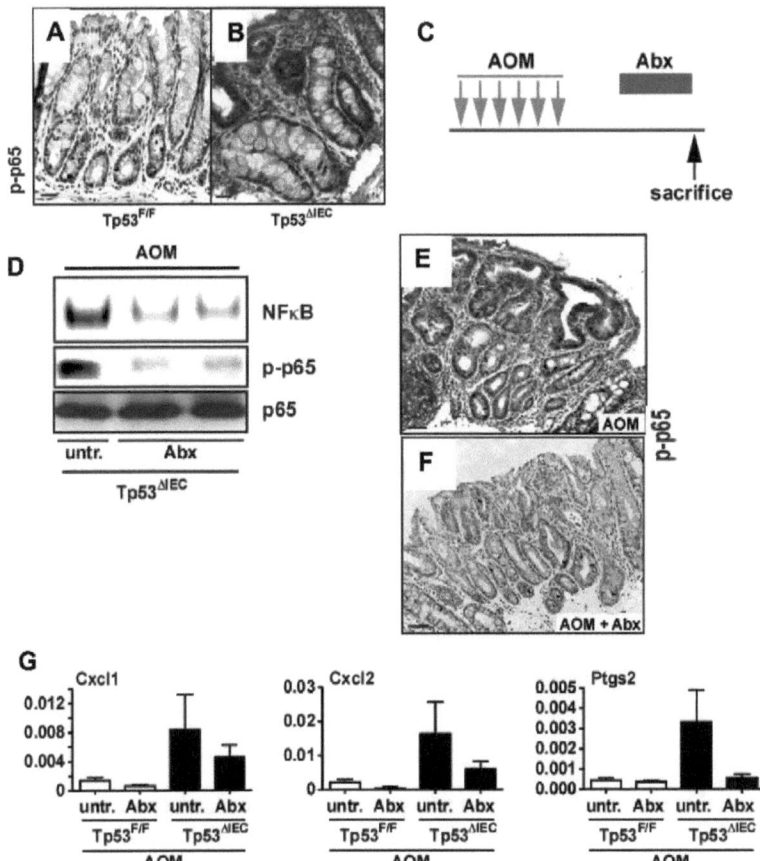

A colored version is available in the electronic edition

Figure 32: Antibiotic treatment of intestinal microbiota results in decreased NF-κB activation in IEC in Tp53$^{\Delta IEC}$ mice

(A, B) Immunohistochemical analysis for phospho- p65 positive epithelial cells in pre-neoplastic colon tissue Tp53$^{F/F}$ and Tp53$^{\Delta IEC}$ mice four weeks after the last AOM challenge. (C) schematic overview depicting the oder of AOM- and antibiotic application. Tp53$^{F/F}$ and Tp53$^{\Delta IEC}$ mice were treated repetitively once a week for 6 weeks with AOM, after two weeks of treatment break an antibiotic cocktail consisting of vancomycin, metronidazole, ampicillin and neomycin (Abx) was given to the animals in the drinking water for 2 weeks prior to sacrifice. (D) EMSA and western blot analysis for NF-κB activity in colon tissue from Tp53$^{\Delta IEC}$ mice with and without antibiotic treatment four weeks after the last AOM application. (E, F) Immunohistochemical analysis for phospho- p65 positive epithelial cells in pre-neoplastic colon tissue of Tp53$^{\Delta IEC}$ mice with and without antibiotic treatment four weeks after the last AOM challenge. (G) relative mRNA expression levels of indicated genes in colon mucosa from antiobiotics treated and untreated Tp53$^{F/F}$ and Tp53$^{\Delta IEC}$ mice 4 weeks after the last AOM application. Data are mean ± SE; n = 6, all data sets are n.s.= not significant; analyzed by one-way ANOVA followed by Bonferroni post hoc test for multiple comparisons (Prism).

3.2.5 IKKβ-dependent NF-κB activation generates a myeloid derived inflammatory microenvironment driving EMT and promotes aggressive tumor invasion and metastatic spread though epithelial Stat3 activation

In order to study the impact of epithelial NF-κB activity on intestinal tumor progression in Tp53$^{\Delta IEC}$ mice, tamoxifen inducible villin-creER^{T2}/Tp53$^{F/F}$ mice were crossed to floxed Ikkβ mice (Ikkβ$^{F/F}$) resulting in an intestinal knockout of IKKβ and p53 after tamoxifen application following AOM challenge (Fig. 33 A). Neither tumor incidence nor apoptosis or proliferation were affected by additional loss of IKKβ in IEC but the number of animals displaying invasive tumors were decreased by 45% and the severity of invasiveness was attenuated as only 10% of invasive tumors invaded the submucosa which was the case in around 30% of Tp53$^{\Delta IEC}$ control mice (Fig. 33 B-F). Accordingly, absence of phosphorylated Ikba and p65 explained decreased Cxcl1 levels (Fig. 34

A, B) and therefore less infiltrated myeloid F4/80+ and Gr1+ cells (Fig 34 C-F). Decreased Twist levels and conversely increased E-Cadherin expression (Fig. 34 G) confirmed that EMT is under control of NF-κB just as it is initiative for the recruitment of inflammatory cells.

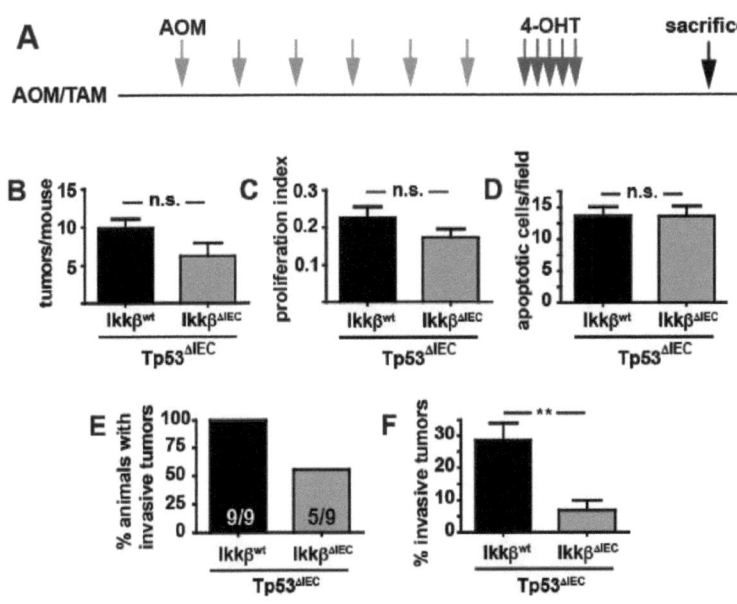

Figure 33: Impaired NF-κB activity results in reduced invasive capability of tumors in Tp53$^{\Delta IEC}$ mice

(A) Schematic depiction of phenotype induction in tamoxifen inducible villin-creER^{T2}/Tp53$^{F/F}$ mice and villin-creER^{T2}/Tp53$^{F/F}$/Ikkβ$^{F/F}$. (B) Tumor incidence in Tp53$^{\Delta IEC}$/Ikkβ^{wt} and Tp53$^{\Delta IEC}$/Ikkβ$^{\Delta IEC}$ mice 18 weeks after tamoxifen administration. Data are mean ± SE; n=9; n.s.: not significant (C) BrdU proliferation index tumor epithelial cells in Tp53$^{\Delta IEC}$/Ikkβ^{wt} and Tp53$^{\Delta IEC}$/Ikkβ$^{\Delta IEC}$ mice. Data are mean ± SE; n≥5 tumors of each genotype; n.s.: not significant (D) Apoptotic index from tumor epithelial cells in Tp53$^{\Delta IEC}$/Ikkβ^{wt} and Tp53$^{\Delta IEC}$/Ikkβ$^{\Delta IEC}$ mice. Data are mean ± SE; n≥5 tumors of each genotype; n.s.: not significant. (E) Proportion of animals in respective indicated genotypes displaying invasive tumors; (F) Percental proportion of invasive tumors per analyzed tumor in all animals Data are mean ± SE; n=9 animals/genotype; ** p < 0.001 by t-test.

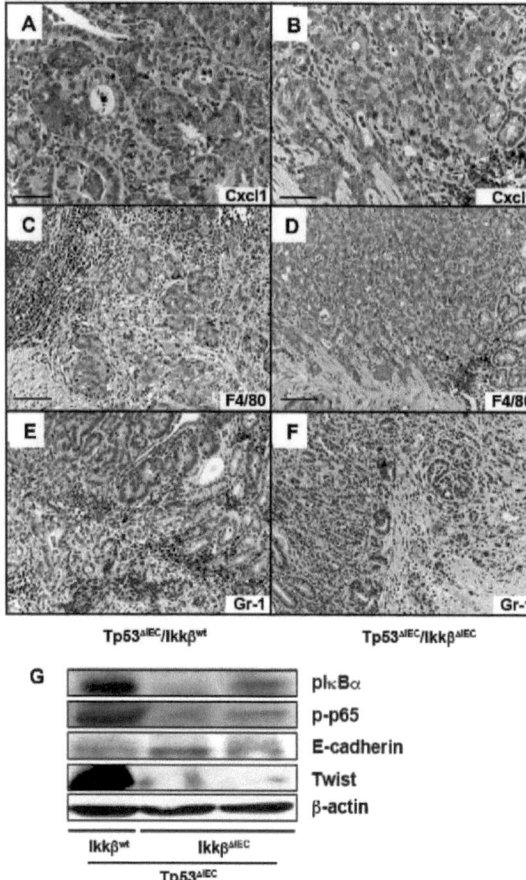

Figure 34: Impaired NF-κB activity results in reduced infiltration of macrophages and neutrophils in tumors of Tp53$^{\Delta IEC}$ mice

Histological analysis of invasive tumors from (A, C, E) Tp53$^{\Delta IEC}$/Ikkβ^{wt} and (B, D, F) Tp53$^{\Delta IEC}$/Ikkβ$^{\Delta IEC}$ mice displaying reduced expression of (A, B) Cxcl1 in IEC and infiltrated cells as well as reduced infiltration of (C, D) F4/80 and (E, F) Gr-1 immune cells in Tp53$^{\Delta IEC}$/Ikkβ$^{\Delta IEC}$ mice. Scale bars = 50 μm. (G) Western blot for EMT markers and NF-κB activation in protein extracts of invasive tumor tissue from Tp53$^{\Delta IEC}$/Ikkβ^{wt} and Tp53$^{\Delta IEC}$/Ikkβ$^{\Delta IEC}$ mice 18 weeks after the first AOM administration.

A colored version is available in the electronic edition

To examine the role of NF-κB in myeloid cells on tumor progression, Tp53$^{\Delta IEC}$ mice were irradiated for lethal depletion of the bone marrow, which was reconstituted with bone marrow from LysM-Cre/Ikkβ$^{F/F}$ or Ikkβ$^{F/F}$ as a control. A direct mating of Tp53$^{\Delta IEC}$ and LysM-Cre/Ikkβ$^{F/F}$ would have resulted in a simultaneous deletion of p53 and IKKβ in myeloid cells as well as IEC. After recovery transplanted animals were treated with AOM to induce tumor development (Fig. 35 A). Tumor incidence as well as invasion incidence were unchanged in comparison to control transplanted Tp53$^{\Delta IEC}$ mice (Fig. 35 B, C), however along the invasive front a decreased proliferation index and increased apoptotic index in IEC became obvious which was associated with a decreased invasive area (Fig. 35 D-F, H, I) and prevention of metastatic spread as no local lymph node metastasis could be detected, while 30% of Tp53$^{\Delta IEC}$ control mice were metastatic (Fig. 35 G). Impaired NF-κB activity in tumor infiltrated myeloid cells resulted in downregulation of crucial tumor promoting factors such as TNFα, IL-1β, IL-11, Cox-2, Cxcl1, Cxcl2, MMP3, MMP10, MMP13 and Cathepsin L in tumors tissues from Tp53$^{\Delta IEC}$ (Fig. 36 A, B), suggesting that infiltrated myeloid cells are responsible for organizing the invasion supporting tumor microenvironment in a NF-κB dependent manner. By means of a colitis associated tumor mouse model it was shown that gp130-dependent Stat3 rather than NF-κB is fundamental for IEC proliferation and tumor progression(Bollrath, Phesse et al. 2009). As markedly decreased expression of IL-11, an activator of Stat3, already suggested, decreased tyrosine-phosphorylated Stat3 was observed in invading tumor cells of Ikkβ$^{\Delta mye}$ transplanted Tp53$^{\Delta IEC}$, while phosphorylation of IκBα was hardly affected (Fig. 36 C- F). Control Tp53$^{\Delta IEC}$ mice however exhibited strong Stat3 activation in IEC along the invasive front and in metastatic IEC, proposing that Stat3, activated through NF-κB dependent myeloid derived microenvironment in a paracrine manner, is crucial for progression of tumor invasion and metastasis formation in Tp53$^{\Delta IEC}$ mice. The correlation of Stat3 activation and the degree of invasion together with the occurrence of lymphatic metastases has been found in studies on human colorectal cancers likewise (Kusaba, Nakayama et al. 2005).

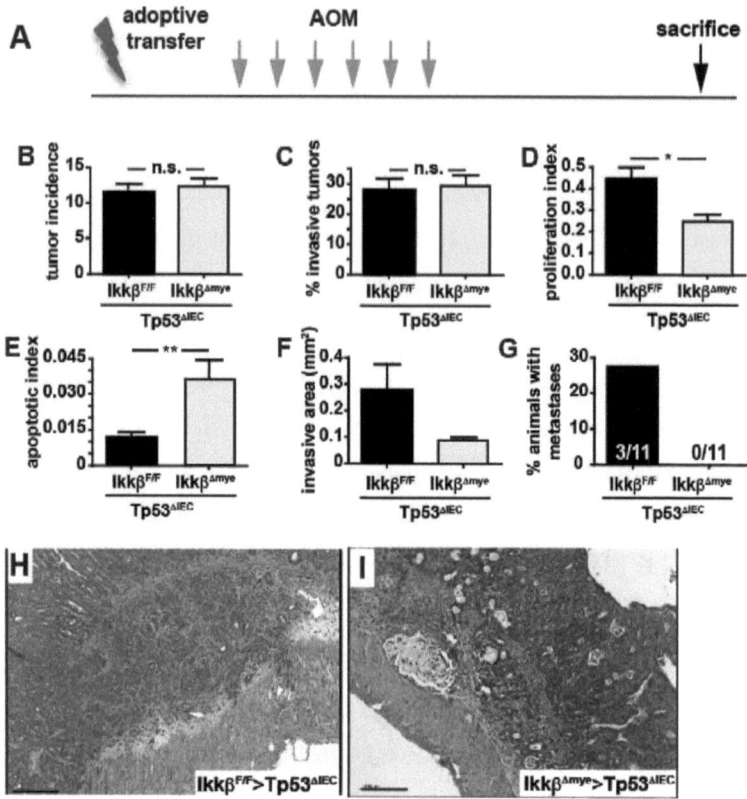

Figure 35: Impaired Ikkβ-dependent NF-κB activation in myeloid cells results in decreased extent of invasion and metastasis formation in tumors of Tp53$^{\Delta IEC}$

(A) Scheme for experimental procedure of the adoptive transfer of bone marrow from Ikkβ$^{F/F}$ or Ikkβ$^{\Delta mye}$ mice injected into lethally irradiated Tp53$^{\Delta IEC}$ animals. After 6 weeks of recovery animals were challenged with AOM. Mice were analyzed 10-13 weeks after first AOM administration. (B) Tumor incidence in AOM treated Tp53$^{\Delta IEC}$ mice transplanted with bone marrow from either Ikkβ$^{\Delta mye}$ or control Ikkβ$^{F/F}$ mice. Data are mean ± SE; n=11 animals; n.s.: not significant. (C) Percental proportion of invasive tumors in either control bone marrow transplanted or Ikkβ$^{\Delta mye}$ transplanted Tp53$^{\Delta IEC}$ mice. Data are mean ± SE; n=11 animals; n.s.: not significant. (D) BrdU proliferation index (D) and cleaved caspase 3 positive cells (E) along the invasion front tumors from Tp53$^{\Delta IEC}$ mice transplanted with Ikkβ$^{F/F}$ or Ikkβ$^{\Delta mye}$ bone marrow. Data are mean ± SE; n≥5 animals;** $p < 0.001$ by t-test. (F) Total invasive tumor area per Ikkβ$^{F/F}$ or Ikkβ$^{\Delta mye}$ bone marrow transplanted Tp53$^{\Delta IEC}$ animal. (G) Metastases incidence in invasive tumor bearing Tp53$^{\Delta IEC}$ mice transplanted with bone marrow from control Ikkβ$^{F/F}$ or Ikkβ$^{\Delta mye}$ mice. (H, I) H&E staining of representative invasive areas in the colon of AOM induced Tp53$^{\Delta IEC}$ mice transplanted with bone marrow from (H) Ikkβ$^{F/F}$ and (I) Ikkβ$^{\Delta mye}$ mice. Scale bars = 200 μm.

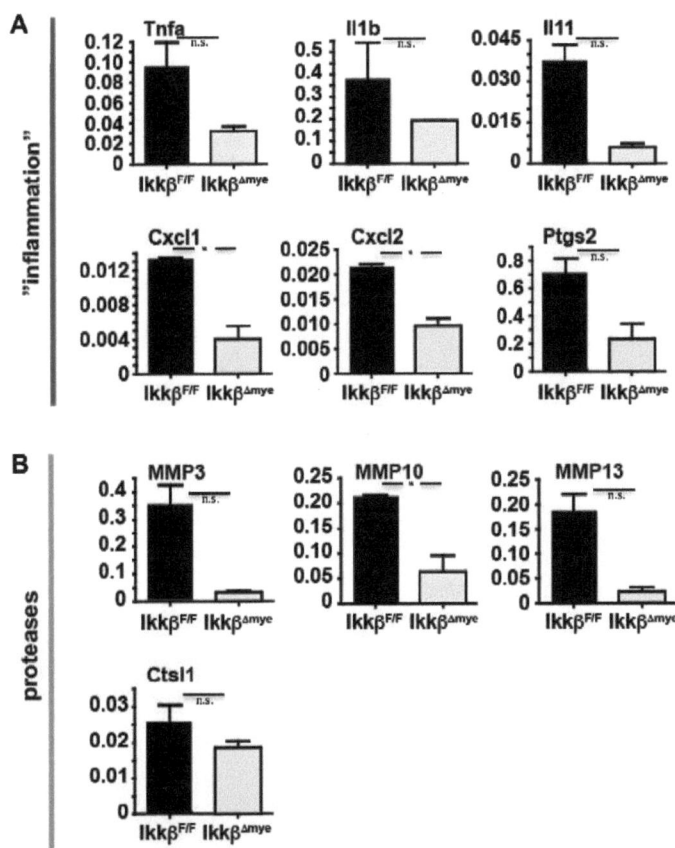

Figure 36: Impaired Ikkβ-dependent NF-κB activation in myeloid cells suppresses the extent of invasion and metastasis formation by failing to activate Stat3 in tumor IEC

(A, B) Relative mRNA expression level of genes belonging functionally to (A) inflammation related markers according to KEGG or to (B) proteases in AOM induced tumor tissue from Tp53ΔIEC mice transplanted with bone marrow from control Ikkβ$^{F/F}$ or Ikkβ$^{\Delta mye}$ mice. Data are mean ± SE; n=2; not indicated data sets are n.s.= not significant; * $p < 0.05$; analyzed by Student's t-test.

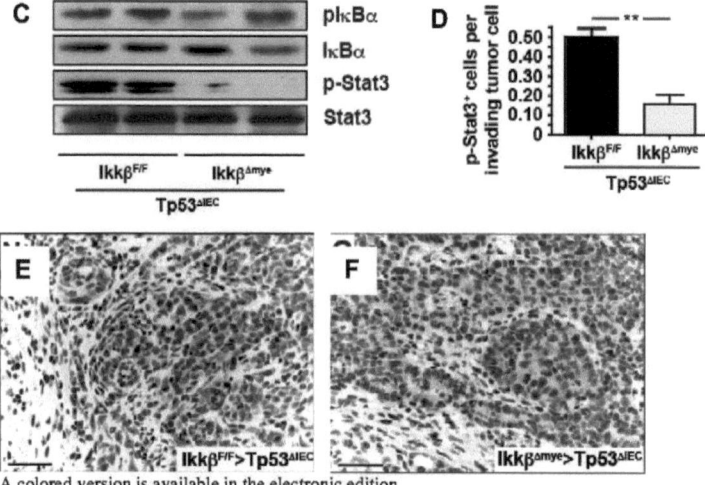

Figure 36: Impaired Ikkβ-dependent NF-κB activation in myeloid cells suppresses the extent of invasion and metastasis formation by failing to activate Stat3 in tumor IEC

(C) Western blot for NF-κB activation or Stat3 activation in invasive cancers from Tp53$^{\Delta IEC}$ mice transplanted with bone marrow from control Ikkβ$^{F/F}$ or Ikkβ$^{\Delta mye}$ mice. (D) Quantification of phosphorylated-Stat3 positive cells/invading tumor epithelial cells in Tp53$^{\Delta IEC}$ mice transplanted with bone marrow from control Ikkβ$^{F/F}$ or Ikkβ$^{\Delta mye}$ mice. Data are mean ± SE; n≥4 animals/genotype; ** p < 0.001 by t-test. (E, F) Immunohistochemistry of phosphorylated Stat3 in invasive tumors of Tp53$^{\Delta IEC}$ mice transplanted with bone marrow from control Ikkβ$^{F/F}$ or Ikkβ$^{\Delta mye}$ mice. Scale bars = 50 μm.

3.2.6 Tp53$^{\Delta IEC}$ mice provide a feasible system for pre-clinical examinations

As Tp53$^{\Delta IEC}$ mice develop tumors in the distal colon resembling the human situation, it is easily possible to detect them by mini-endoscopy (Becker, Fantini et al. 2006) (Fig. 37 A, B). Therefore Tp53$^{\Delta IEC}$ mice might represent a reasonable *in vivo* system for pre-clinical studies. For example, by miniprobe based confocal laser scanning microscopy (CLSM) after intravenous application of fluorescein it is possible to detect changes in the vascularization in different tumor stages (Waldner, Wirtz et al. 2011). According to the angiogenic switch hypothesis (Bergers and Benjamin 2003) and as detection of augmented hypoxic (Fig. 37 H-J) areas depending on the tumor stage suggests, indeed a significant increase of blood vessel length and blood vessel area from early to late stage carcinogenesis could be visualized by CLSM in Tp53$^{\Delta IEC}$ mice (Fig. 37 E, F) which was confirmed by immunohistochemical VE-Cadherin vessel quantification (Fig. 37 G). In humans CLSM has already been applied successfully in Barrett's esophagus as well as for the diagnosis of biliary neoplasia (Meining, Frimberger et al. 2008; Pohl, Rosch et al. 2008). Moreover, upon treatment with the anti- angiogenic receptor tyrosine kinase inhibitor sunitinib, CLSM confirmed a significant decrease in vessel length and area in tumor bearing Tp53$^{\Delta IEC}$ mice (Fig. 37 L, M). Therefore, the possibility for using CLSM in mice opens up an avenue for detecting the success of anti-angiogenic therapies and supports the suitability of the mouse model for pre-clinical studies.

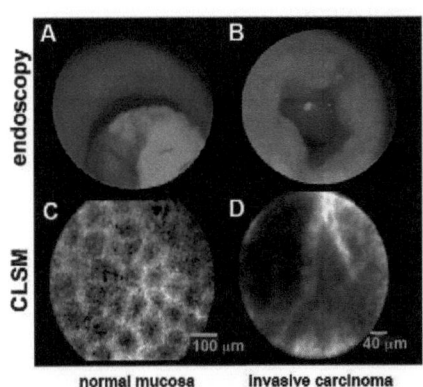
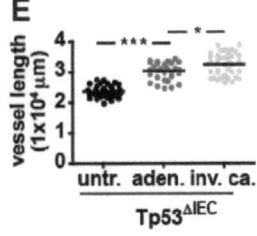

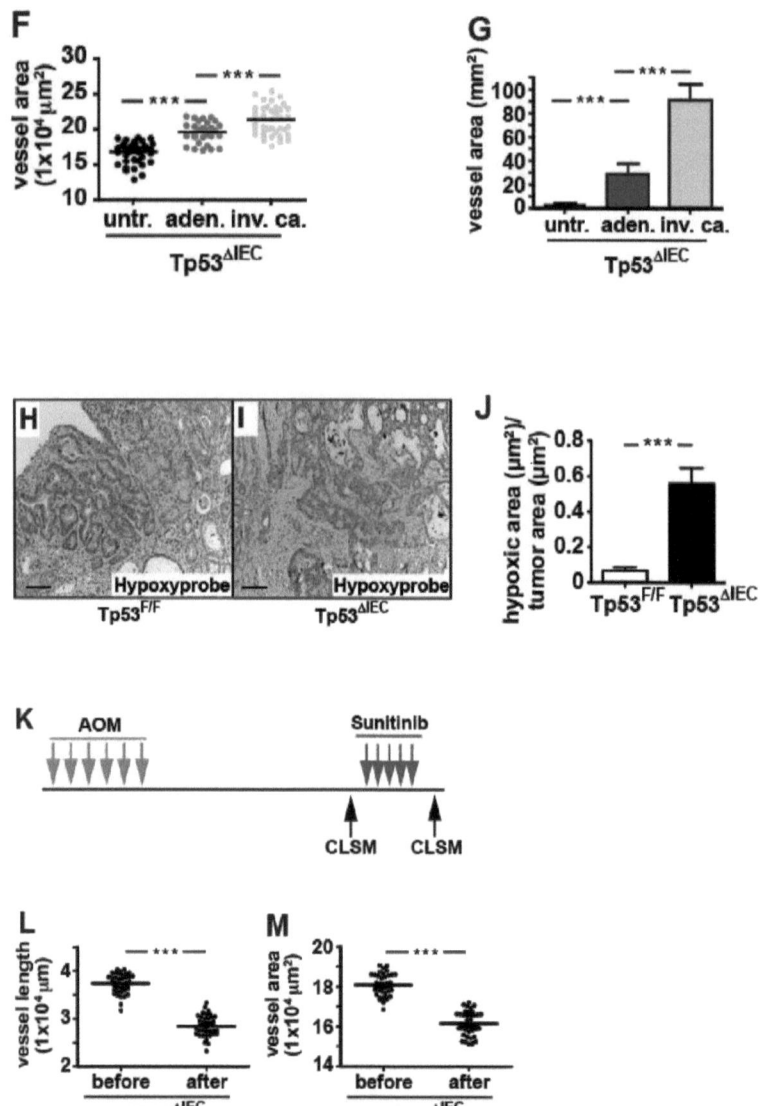

A colored version is available in the electronic edition

Figure 37: AOM induced Tp53$^{\Delta IEC}$ mice as a suitable pre-clinical model for therapies

(A, B) Detection of (B) distal colonic tumors in AOM-induced Tp53$^{\Delta IEC}$ mice in advanced and invasive tumor stage compared to (A) unchallenged animals. (C, D)

Detection of vessel structure by confocal laser scanning microscopy (clsm) in (C) unchallenged and (D) Tp53$^{\Delta IEC}$ mice with invasive cancer after intravenous fluorescein injection. (E) Quantification of blood vessel length and (F) blood vessel area (F) in untreated (untr.) animals, non-invasive (aden.) and invasive tumors (inv. ca.) in Tp53$^{\Delta IEC}$ mice analyzed using IC viewer software for Cellvizio® imager (Mauna Kea Tech). Data are mean ± SE; n ≥ 4. *** p < 0.0001 and * p < 0.05 analyzed by one-way ANOVA followed by Bonferroni post hoc test for multiple comparisons (G) Quantification of blood vessel area by means of VE-Cadherin immunohistochemically stained vessels in untreated animals, non-invasive and invasive cancers in Tp53$^{\Delta IEC}$ mice analyzed on a Zeiss Axio Imager using AxioVision software. Data are mean ± SE; n ≥ 6; *** p < 0.0001 analyzed by one-way ANOVA followed by Bonferroni post hoc test for multiple comparisons. (H, I) Immunohistochemical hypoxia visualization using Hypoxyprobe showing (I) enlarged hypoxic areas in tumors from Tp53$^{\Delta IEC}$ mice compared to (H) noninvasive adenoma from Tp53$^{F/F}$ mice. (J) Quantification of hypoxic areas per tumor area in non-invasive adenomas from Tp53$^{F/F}$ mice and invasive cancers from Tp53$^{\Delta IEC}$ mice 16 weeks after the first AOM administration. Data are mean ± SE; n ≥ 4; *** p < 0.0001 by t-test. (K) Schematic overview for the application of the anti- angiogenic therapeutical Sunitinib during the late tumor stages of AOM-induced Tp53$^{\Delta IEC}$ mice and detection of changes in the tumor vascularization by performing CLSM. (L) Quantification of blood vessel length and (M) blood vessel area by CLSM after fluorescein injection in tumors of Tp53$^{\Delta IEC}$ mice before and after Sunitinib treatment. Data are mean ± SE; n ≥ 4. *** p < 0.0001 by t-test.

4. Discussion

4.1 NF-κB can be activated by diverse mechanisms and in turn modulates Wnt signaling by direct crosstalk with β-catenin during tumor initiation

Inflammation is linked clinically and epidemiologically to cancer and NF-κB activation appears to play a causative role, but the mechanisms are poorly understood. Meta-analyses document a significant decrease in colorectal tumor incidence and tumor burden in humans after long-term preventative administration of non-steroidal anti-inflammatory drugs such as Aspirin (Chan, Ogino et al. 2009; Rothwell, Fowkes et al. 2011) which is shown to specifically inhibit IKKβ activity *in vitro* and *in vivo* (Yin, Yamamoto et al. 1998), thus assigning NF-κB a role already during the earliest steps of the tumorigenic process, but mechanistic proof *in vivo* was still missing until now.

Above data demonstrate that NF-κB modulates aberrant Wnt signaling during tumor initiation by enhancing the binding of β-catenin to the promoters of intestinal stem cell target genes and therefore accelerates the formation of a crypt progenitor phenotype and malignant transformation.

Interestingly, in Helicobacter pylori–induced gastric tumors, NF-κB signaling induced by tumor necrosis factor Tnf-α can induce β-catenin nuclear accumulation even without the presence of APC mutations (Oguma, Oshima et al. 2008). Analogously, production of prostaglandin E2 (PGE2) by cyclooxygenase 2 (COX2) during acute and chronic inflammation induced by NF-κB and Akt pathway activity, also increases β-catenin nuclear accumulation (Castellone, Teramoto et al. 2005; Kaler, Augenlicht et al. 2009; Kaler, Godasi et al. 2009) furthermore underscoring the power of NF-κB in promoting tumorigenesis even in the absence of preceding Wnt component mutations.

A direct cross- talk between NF-κB and β-catenin has already been suggested for several tumor cell lines, albeit with different effects (Spiegelman, Slaga et al. 2000; Deng, Miller et al. 2002). In a colon cancer cell line it was observed that β-catenin inhibits NF-κB activity (Deng, Miller et al. 2002), however above data demonstrate a direct physical interaction of NF-κB, activated by either autocrine or paracrine secreted Tnf-α, and mutant β-catenin via recruitment of co-factor CBP in IEC *in vivo*. Elevated NF-κB activity accelerated malignant transformation by promoting strengthened binding of β-catenin to its target genes and consequently enhanced expression of stem cell signature genes (Fig. 39). Furthermore, data point out that NF-κB activity can also be increased by oncogenic K-Ras in primary IEC (Fig 13). Supportingly, oncogenic K-Ras activity was recently shown to activate NF-κB in a mouse model of pancreatic ductal adenocarcinoma (PDAC) (Ling, Kang et al. 2012). Furthermore, oncogenic K-Ras activity has been found before to correlate with oncogenic Wnt signaling in human cell lines and human FAP patients (Wu, Tu et al. 2008; Phelps, Chidester et al. 2009). Moreover, in a cohort of CRC patients with oncogenic K-Ras activation a specific gene expression pattern indicated a crosstalk of mutant K-Ras with Wnt and NF-κB pathways (Watanabe, Kobunai et al. 2011).

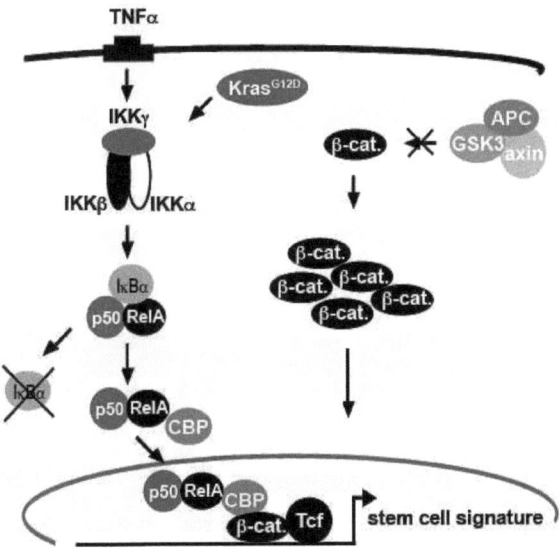

Figure 38: Representative scheme modeling the mechanism of NF-κB triggered Wnt dependent cell transformation

IKKβ-dependent NF-κB activation is induced by TNFα or oncogenic K-Ras and the signaling complex further recruits the common co-activator CBP. In the nucleus the complex enhances binding of β-catenin to respective promoter sequences to promote transcription of Wnt-dependent stem cell genes.

Additionally, in collaboration with O. Sansom it was demonstrated that

NF-κB activation depends on the activity of the GTPase Rac1. In a mouse model with intestinal deletion of the Wnt pathway component APC Rac1 is activated downstream of Wnt activity and induces the production of reactive oxygen species (ROS) which in turn activate NF-κB and supports formation of a crypt progenitor phenotype and subsequent tumorigenesis. However, upon deletion of Rac1 hyperproliferation was stopped and the crypt progenitor phenotype reversed underscoring the necessity of NF-κB activity for modulation of Wnt regulated intestinal stem cell signature (Myant et al., in revision 2012).

4.2 NF-κB patronizes cell type plasticity during tumor initiation and during tumor progression

Interestingly, intensified Wnt signaling triggered by enhanced NF-κB activation resulted in re-expression of stem cell markers even in differentiated enterocytes (Fig. 11,13) leading to the formation of aberrant crypt foci in the villus compartment, apart from the accepted "bottom-up" concept of transformed crypt stem cells which states that Lgr5+ crypt stem cells are the cell-of-origin for intestinal tumor development and has been proven *in vivo* recently (Barker, Ridgway et al. 2009). Re-expression of the multipotent stem cell marker Lgr5+ in above shown de novo formed crypts and in tumors arising from differentiated epithelial cells gives proof of principle that de-differentiation is a feasible event in tumor initiation. This finding corroborates the "top-down" theory of tumorigenesis claiming that transformed, dysplastic cells spread laterally and downwards to form new crypts (Shih, Wang et al. 2001), which is in contrast yet does not exclude the "bottom-up" concept Barker et al. proved *in vivo* likewise (Fig. 39).

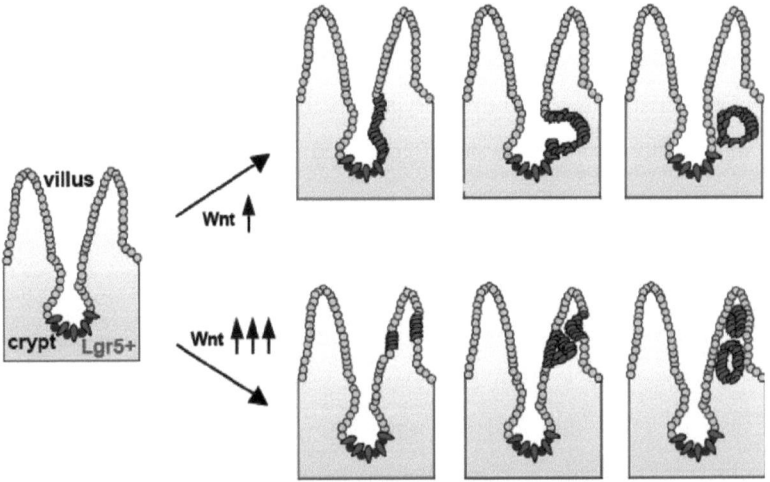

Figure 39: Schematic overview of the "Bottom-up" and "Top-down" cell-of-origin concept for the intestinal tumorigenesis

The "bottom-up" model (Oshima, Oshima et al. 1997) takes affect predominantly when a normal mode of aberrant Wnt activation after loss of Apc or activating mutations of Ctnnb result in adenomatous transformation of Lgr5+ stem cells at the bottom of the crypt (red) and their invagination into the subepithelium. The "top-down" concept applies in case of strongly enhanced aberrant Wnt signaling leading to dedifferentiation of enterocytes and reexpression of stem cell marker Lgr5+ conferring initially differentiated cells the same tumorigenic potential as crypt stem cells.

Recently, dysfunction of pancreatic b-cells resulting in type 2 diabetes has been shown to be associated with FoxO1 dependent dedifferentiation of b-cells to uncommitted endocrine progenitor cells *in vivo* and even conversion of b-cells into other hormone producing pancreatic cells (Talchai, Xuan et al. 2012). Even though to a limited extent, the process of de-differentiation has also been observed to occur in mouse differentiating spermatogonia that converted to germinal stem cells *in vivo* (Barroca, Lassalle et al. 2009) and moreover in basal-like mammary epithelial cells spontaneously converting into cancer stem cell like cells *in vitro* (Chaffer, Brueckmann et al. 2011). *Ex vivo* de-differentiated transformed villus epithelial cells from $APC^{DIEC}Kras^{G12D}$ mice injected into nude mice demonstrated tumor growth with similar growth characteristics as transformed crypt cells from $APC^{DIEC}Kras^{G12D}$ mice and importantly tumors from de-differentiated villus epithelial cells were re-expressing stem cell marker Lgr5 proving that de-differentiated epithelial cells are able to give rise to tumor initiating cells. Furthermore, serial transplantations and serial dilutions of de-differentiated transformed villus cells into nude mice demonstrated even the generation of cancer stem cells (CSCs) from differentiated cells (Schwitalla et al.). Above findings of de-differentiation and CSC generation are supported by observations made in recent lineage tracing experiments showing that CSCs arise de novo during tumor formation in intact organs (Chen, Li et al. 2012; Driessens, Beck et al. 2012) which sheds new light on the hitherto understanding of cell commitment and tumor cell hierarchies stating that tumor stem cells spawn more highly differentiated cells in solid tumors. Regarding the depicted *in vivo* proof of dedifferentiation and similar hints throughout the literature it seems conceivable in general that non-stem cells can be reversed to a stem-cell-like state either by caused mutations, or even spontaneously (Gupta, Fillmore et al. 2011) and so contribute to tumor evolution. Importantly, similar observations were also made in human tissue sections from a cohort of ulcerative colitis patients (Schwitalla et al. 2013) in which in situ hybridizations revealed strong expression of the stem cell marker OLFM4 in epithelial cell entities at the margin of the ulcus suggesting that these aberrant crypt foci formed de novo by de-differentiation even in the absence of oncogenic mutations supporting the significance of chronic inflammatory conditions and the microenvironment for de-differentiation based cell transformation and increased colorectal cancer incidence in humans as well.

Cell type plasticity is expected to occur not only during tumor initiation (Fig.13) but also in tumor cells converting to invading and metastasizing CSCs through epithelial-mesenchymal-transition (EMT) during the course of tumor progression (Brabletz, Jung et al. 2005; Thiery and Sleeman 2006). The reprogramming is supposed to be mediated by microenvironmental signals (Gupta, Chaffer et al. 2009; Rosen and Jordan 2009; Vermeulen, De Sousa et al. 2010; Medema and Vermeulen 2011). Of note, the de-differentiation process neither during tumor initiation (Fig. 13) nor implicated during EMT (Fig. 18) is observed by solely stabilizing b-catenin or by disrupting APC (Barker, Ridgway et al. 2009) unless modulating factors such as NF-κB, activated by Tnf-α or oncogenic K-Ras, trigger the process by enhancing Wnt activity even further. The fact that NF-κB interferes with transcription of stem cell markers, regulates the expression of EMT markers such as Twist in p53 deficient cells and is responsible for the creation of an EMT supporting inflammatory microenvironment (Fig. 18) underscores the conciseness of NF-κB on all steps during carcinogenesis, on the one hand during tumor initiation by enabling de-differentiation and therefore enlarging the pool of transformed cells, on the other hand during tumor progression by triggering EMT via trans-differentiation of tumor cells which leave the primary tumor site in order to give rise to metastatic spread accounting for a poor prognosis in patients (Ignatiadis, Rothe et al. 2011; Sanger, Effenberger et al. 2011). NF-κB may also influence development and promotion of de-differentiated tumor cells up to CSC formation by directly controlling the expression of even pluripotency factors such as Lin28, which is shown to be a component of the reprogramming transcription factor cocktail to generate induced pluripotent stem cells (iPSCs) (Yu, Vodyanik et al. 2007). Recently it has been shown in human immortalized breast cells, wich developed self-renewing spheres containing cancer stem cells, that NF-κB directly activates Lin28 transcription and rapidly reduces let-7 micro-RNA levels, normally known to inhibit IL6 expression, resulting in higher levels of IL6 than achieved by NF-κB activation. IL6- activates STAT3 and further NF-κB, thereby completing a positive feedback loop. This regulatory circuit operates in other cancer cell lines, and its transcriptional signature is also found in human cancer tissues (Iliopoulos, Hirsch et al. 2009). Thus, NF-κB induced inflammatory conditions activate a positive feedback loop that can maintain the transformed state for many generations even in the absence of the inducing signal.

Consequently, NF-κB seems to influence a dynamic equilibrium between more or less differentiated tumor cells and CSCs as well as transformed differentiated cells and has the ability to provoke an equilibrium shift in favor of tumor initiating cells or tumor fuelling CSCs. Above demonstrated data give evidence that de-differentiation is de facto a certain event critically underestimated so far, as the idea questions the unidirectional, hierarchical model of cell development and cell commitment. Cell type plasticity during tumor initiation and within tumor tissue strikes a new path from strict cell undirectionality towards bidirectional interconversion resulting in a dynamic equilibrium of cell populations which might complicate therapeutic strategies. Selectively killing CSCs may vacate a niche within the tumor, opening it up to occupancy by a rival population of cells underlying de-differentiation. Although targeting both CSCs and their daughter cells with a combination of suicide-gene targeting and anticancer drugs dramatically impeded the growth of glioblastomas in *in vivo* mouse models (Chen, Li et al. 2012), an even more effective way rather than simply eradicating

CSCs and the tumor bulk may be destroying the CSC promoting niche by educating the tumor microenvironment.

4.3 Indirect inverse crosstalk between NF-κB and p53 function reveals differing tissue specific tumor suppressive roles of p53 during tumor initiation and tumor progression

It is demonstrated above that the NF-κB dependent pro-inflammatory microenvironment aggravates tumor invasion by further activating Stat3 in invading tumor cells and thereby promoting survival and proliferation of the invasive tumors culminating in lymph node metastasis (Fig. 15). Tumor cells gained invasive capability by becoming a subject to cell type plasticity through NF-κB controlled EMT marker expression. Moreover, a decisive genetic event enabling colorectal tumor progression is the loss of the tumor suppressive function of p53 as 100% of TP53$^{\Delta IEC}$ mice displayed invasive tumor growth albeit only after enforcing additional mutations in the Wnt pathway by carcinogenic challenge. This fact underlines the requirement of certain mutations to progress tumorigenesis which supports the step-wise model of colorectal carcinogenesis (Fearon and Vogelstein 1990). According to above data p53's tumor suppressive role in Wnt-driven tumorigenesis can be specified as the "guardian of invasiveness" rather than being implicated in the well established cell-autonomous functions such apoptosis induction, cell cycle arrest and senescence (Junttila and Evan 2009). The invasiveness control by p53 during Wnt driven tumorigenesis has also been found in a CK1-α/p53 intestinal double knockout mouse model, however by the regulation of a p53-suppressed invasiveness gene signature (PSIS) rather than by the classic EMT process (Elyada, Pribluda et al. 2011) contrasting the dependence of invasion on NF-κB regulated EMT marker expression in

TP53$^{\Delta IEC}$ mice (Fig. 18) and other similar observations in p53 mutant cell lines directly regulating EMT (Wang, Wang et al. 2009). Furthermore, TP53$^{\Delta IEC}$ colonic tumors did not display a significant enrichment of PSIS genes, which could be attributed to a differentially activated aberrant Wnt pathway or due to the location of the tumors in the colon rather than in the small intestine, which can affect the mode of NF-κB activation.

During tumor initiation the TP53^{DIEC} mouse model revealed a supplementary role for p53 as it controls apoptosis and DNA damage repair of AOM affected cells which is in accordance with its already investigated function as the guardian of the genome (Lane 1992) in terms of genotoxic injury response (Meek 2009). The important tumor suppressor function of p53 is well established for several types of solid tumors (Blons and Laurent-Puig 2003; Iacopetta 2003; Schuijer and Berns 2003) of which an abundant proportion of up to 70% showed somatic p53 mutations correlating with malignancy while only ~ 10% of hematopoietic malignancies revealed a loss of p53 function (Peller and Rotter 2003). Supportingly, the suppression of radiation- induced lymphoma by p53 in mice was dispensable and was carried out by a p53-independent mechanism (Christophorou, Ringshausen et al. 2006). Altogether these findings suggest a tissue specific tumor suppressive role for p53. The specificity for colon tissue is especially given by the fact that p53 loss results in an intestinal epithelial barrier defect, which is highly pronounced upon carcinogen exposure, leading to enhanced attachment of intestinal bacteria and increased serum LPS levels which induce NF-κB activity (Fig. 21) required for progressing invasion. Therefore data indicate that p53 indirectly suppresses the recruitment of a pro-inflammatory microenvironment by preventing endotoxin caused NF-κB activation. Correlation between mutant nonfunctional p53 and NF-κB was shown in cancer cells as well although in a direct dependence of mutant p53 and enhanced NF-κB response to TNF-α (Weisz, Damalas et al. 2007), and transcriptionally activated NFKB2 (Scian, Stagliano et al. 2005) suggesting that Tp53 mutations might activate the pro-inflammatory NF-κB pathway and promote tumorigenesis in the context of chronic inflammation as well.

4.4 Intestinal microbiata has a unique tissue specific tumor promoting role

The loss of p53 in IEC resulted in the development of an carcinogen induced intestinal barrier defect during tumor development and subsequent enhanced epithelial NF-κB activation caused by endotoxins from the intestinal microflora promoting EMT and the recruitment of a tumor microenvrionment.

Of note, the indirect inverse cross- talk between p53 function and p65 activity upon carcinogen exposure *in vivo* confers p53 a new tissue specific involvement in epithelial barrier protection and concomitantly highlights the contribution of intestinal microflora to support colorectal tumorigenesis even in spontaneous CRC. It is conceivable that after carcinogen exposure intestinal cell adhesion complexes and epithelial barrier composition is changed due to a shift of carcinogenically mutated β-catenin from membranous/cytoplasmic to nuclear localization and is therefore more susceptible to develop an epithelial barrier defect in combination with p53 loss of function even during early stages of tumorigenesis which becomes more pronounced upon further tumor growth. As the tumor cells expand and the tumor structure changes cell adhesion contacts are further reorganized and enhanced intestinal permeability is even more aggravated in p53 loss-of-function IEC enabling the attachment and infiltration of intestinal bacteria and subsequent NF-κB activation triggering EMT expression, which proposes a direct or indirect cross talk between cell adhesion/tight junction signaling and p53 function. Formerly it was found that integrin signaling related focal adhesion kinase (FAK) is able to bind and suppress p53 and induces proliferation and cell survival during wound healing after DSS-induced colitis in the colon of mice (Golubovskaya and Cance 2011; Owen, Abshire et al. 2011). Other scenarios of p53 interacting with other cell adhesion/tight junction complex members and vice versa or even transcriptional and/or translational control of tight junction proteins by p53 are supposable likewise after carcinogenic challenge.

In the context of chronic inflammatory conditions it is well established that the intestinal microbiota plays a key role in the pathogenesis of Crohn's disease (CD) and ulcerative colitis (UC) collectively referred to as inflammatory bowel disease (IBD). Epidemiological studies have provided strong evidence that IBD patients bear increased risk for the development of colorectal cancer (CRC) (Itzkowitz and Harpaz 2004; Rutter, Saunders et al. 2004; Gupta, Harpaz et al. 2007), but the mechanisms remain elusive. By modulating the content of intestinal bacteria it was shown that AOM-treated $Il10^{-/-}$ mice develop colon cancer in the presence of colitogenic bacteria whereas germ-free mice remain disease-free. Additionally, AOM-treated $Il10^{-/-}/Myd88^{-/-}$ mice failed to develop colorectal tumors suggesting that bacterial signaling through the TLR/MyD88 system is required for development of colitis associated colon cancer (CAC) (Uronis, Muhlbauer et al. 2009). Recently it was reported that conversely inflammation targets the microbiota to foster the expansion of bacteria with genotoxic potential (Arthur, Perez-Chanona et al. 2012) and to adhere to the colonic mucosa by decreasing protective mucins and antimicrobial peptide production (Schwerbrock, Makkink et al. 2004; Inaba, Ashida et al. 2010), so genotoxic bacteria can readily access the epithelium. This suggests that not only enhanced influence of commensal microbiota in terms of increased bacterial population or enhanced attachment but also a microflora shift during the course of tumor development leading to overgrowth of genotoxic or pathogenic counterparts eventually induced by the inflammatory tumor microenvironment or even by the tumor itself can negatively favor carcinogenesis. Due to these findings one has to take into account that the luminal bacteria might be a pivotal modifiable risk factor for individualized interventions. Current initiatives, such as the NIH-funded human microbiome project help to increase the knowledge about the intricate relationship between the microflora and host (Peterson, Garges et al. 2009).

4.5 The TP53$^{\Delta IEC}$ mouse model represents the human course of colorectal cancer and is a suitable model for pre-clinical studies

Upon carcinogenic challenge which induces activating mutations in the Ctnnb gene TP53$^{\Delta IEC}$ mice developed invasive and metastasizing distal colorectal tumors and hence displayed the whole spectrum of the colorectal tumorigenic course from initial neoplastic lesions and adenoma growth up to invasive carcinoma and metastases formation. Tumorigenesis in TP53$^{\Delta IEC}$ mice was majorly accompanied by an NF-κB dependent inflammatory microenvironment supporting the similarity to human colorectal cancer and the assignability of reported findings in mice to the human situation.

To date there are merely few mouse models that develop spontaneous colonic tumors and even metastasis according to Fearon and Vogelstein's genetic model of colorectal tumorigenesis comparing the classic adenoma-carcinoma-metastasis axis found in humans. Representing the variety of human APC mutations, mouse strains containing different types of truncated APC gene have been generated displaying subtle differences in location and number of the adenomas depending on the dosage of Wnt signaling (Aoki, Tamai et al. 2003). A compromising mutation in the colon epithelial cell differentiation regulator Cdx2 in APC^{Min} mice results in a shift of adenomatous non-invasive polyps to the colon (Aoki, Tamai et al. 2003). A deletion of the tumor suppressor Pten in APC^{Min} mice however led to more dysplasia and enhanced invasive growth in the small intestine (Marsh, Winton et al. 2008). As 50% of human colorectal tumors develop oncogenic KRAS activating mutations promoting tumor progression, several mouse models have been developed in which mutationally inactivated APC and simultaneous oncogenic K-Ras activation showed tumor progression including invasive capabilities in the colon and liver metastasis (Janssen, Alberici et al. 2006; Sansom, Meniel et al. 2006; Haigis, Kendall et al. 2008; Luo, Brooks et al. 2009; Hung, Maricevich et al. 2010). In contrast carcinogen challenged TP53^{ΔIEC} mice did not develop K-Ras mutations per se and oncogenic K-Ras activation does not necessarily lead to tumor invasion upon AOM exposure (Bennecke, Kriegl et al. 2010) further underlining the necessity for further genetic alterations leading to p53 function disruption and concomitant NF-κB activity enabling EMT and recruitment of the proinflammatory microenvironment. Indeed, in human colorectal tumors obtained from a patient cohort there was a significant correlation between p53 mutations, phosphorylated nuclear p65 and infiltration of CD68 positive macrophages (Fig. 18). 30 % of the

TP53^{DIEC} mice developed lymph node metastasis furthermore resembling the human course as lymph node metastasis occurence was found to be correlating with Cxcl-1 and Twist expression (Valdes-Mora, Gomez del Pulgar et al. 2009; Ogata, Sekikawa et al. 2010) and with NF- κB activation in human patients (Fig. 18).

A tumorigenic course comparable to humans, distal colorectal location of tumors and its immunocompetence suggests the TP53^{DIEC} mouse model to be one of the most suitable *in vivo* systems, rather than xenograft models (Ellis and Fidler 2010), to study genetic alterations, microenvironmental impact as well as aberrant cell signaling in order to unravel the mechanisms behind tumor progression, namely invasion and metastases formation. Xenograft mouse models do not reflect the sporadic nature of colon cancer and do not allow the investigation of the pro- or antitumorigenic impact of the inflammatory microenvironment due to the lack of a natural recruitment of immune cells induced by secreted factors from tumor cells. The observation of inflammatory cells in pre-malignant tissue, seen as „wounds that do not heal" (Dvorak 1986) and further the presence of inflammatory infiltrate in and around developed tumors facilitating tumor invasion and metastatic spread (Fig. 28) supports the urgent necessity to study the micronvironmental crosstalk with tumor cells *in vivo* which is solely enabled by using an immunocompetent mouse model. Apart from a naturally developing NF-κB dependent inflammatory microenvironment, the immunocompetent TP53^{DIEC} mouse model also offered the advantage of examining the tissue specific tumor suppressive function of p53 and revealed the impact of another tissue specific tumor promoting component, the intestinal microbiota, which merely would have been possible using a xenograft model.

Furthermore the possibility of endoscopic tumor detection in the TP53$^{\Delta IEC}$ mouse model renders it to be interesting for pre-clinical investigations. Of note, it was possible to readily monitor and quantitatively assess the positive efficacy of the anti-angiogenic effects of sunitinib, originally applied in human renal cell carcinoma and in gastrointestinal stromal tumor patients, predicting a confident outcome if applied in human colorectal cancer patients as well and opens up a promising avenue for a positive benefit using other tumor targeting therapeutics.

Summary

Persistent activation of NF-κB has been observed in a variety of tumor tissues including colorectal cancer but its specific function is only poorly understood. In order to study the influence of NF-κB on different stages of intestinal tumorigenesis, diverse genetic mouse models were used. One of the first steps during tumor initiation is attributed to mutations in the Wnt pathway. By means of a mouse model having an epithelial specific mutation in the Ctnnb gene leading to a constitutively active Wnt pathway and crypt stem cell expansion, NF-κB was shown to modulate aberrant Wnt signaling by modifying stem cell target gene transcription on the promoter level. While deletion of NF-κB delays cell transformation, conversely enhanced NF-κB activity promoted the phenotype and resulted in the formation of foci displaying stem cell characteristics in aberrant position. This observation supports the notion that post-mitotic cells can dedifferentiate *in vivo* to acquire tumor-initiating properties. Generating a new transgenic mouse model allowing recombination in non-stem cells only confirmed this hypothesis.

During the course of tumor development additional mutations in oncogenes or tumor suppressive genes such as Tp53 are required for tumor progression. Although loss of p53 in intestinal epithelial cells alone was not sufficient to initiate intestinal tumorigenesis, however challenge with the carcinogen AOM, causing additional Wnt activation, resulted in increased tumor incidence and spontaneous colorectal invasive tumor growth including lymph node metastasis. After carcinogen exposure p53 controlled DNA damage and IEC survival, while during invasive tumor growth, loss of p53 was associated with increased intestinal permeability causing formation of an NF-κB dependent inflammatory microenvironment and the induction of epithelial-mesenchymal transition regulated by NF-κB. This suggests different roles of p53 during tumor initiation and during tumor progression and confers p53 a novel tissue specific tumor suppressive role as guardian of invasiveness apart from its well-established role in cell cycle regulation, apoptosis and senescence.

This work highlights the celltype and context specific functions of NF-κB during intestinal tumorigenesis as NF-κB is demonstrated to be substantially involved in cell type plasticity during tumor initiation and tumor invasion and is responsible for the recruitment of an inflammatory microenvironment.

Citation Index

Aggarwal, B. B. (2004). "Nuclear factor-kappaB: the enemy within." Cancer Cell 6(3): 203-208.

Al-Hajj, M., M. S. Wicha, et al. (2003). "Prospective identification of tumorigenic breast cancer cells." Proc Natl Acad Sci U S A 100(7): 3983-3988.

Algul, H., M. Treiber, et al. (2007). "Pancreas-specific RelA/p65 truncation increases susceptibility of acini to inflammation-associated cell death following cerulein pancreatitis." J Clin Invest 117(6): 1490-1501.

Aoki, K., Y. Tamai, et al. (2003). "Colonic polyposis caused by mTOR-mediated chromosomal instability in Apc+/Delta716 Cdx2+/- compound mutant mice." Nat Genet 35(4): 323-330.

Araki, Y., S. Okamura, et al. (2003). "Regulation of cyclooxygenase-2 expression by the Wnt and ras pathways." Cancer Res 63(3): 728-734.

Archbold, H. C., Y. X. Yang, et al. (2012). "How do they do Wnt they do?: regulation of transcription by the Wnt/beta-catenin pathway." Acta Physiol (Oxf) 204(1): 74-109.

Arthur, J. C., E. Perez-Chanona, et al. (2012). "Intestinal Inflammation Targets Cancer-Inducing Activity of the Microbiota." Science.

Ashton-Rickardt, P. G., M. G. Dunlop, et al. (1989). "High frequency of APC loss in sporadic colorectal carcinoma due to breaks clustered in 5q21-22." Oncogene 4(10): 1169-1174.

Aspord, C., A. Pedroza-Gonzalez, et al. (2007). "Breast cancer instructs dendritic cells to prime interleukin 13-secreting CD4+ T cells that facilitate tumor development." J Exp Med 204(5): 1037-1047.

Barker, N., R. A. Ridgway, et al. (2009). "Crypt stem cells as the cells-of-origin of intestinal cancer." Nature 457(7229): 608-611.

Barker, N., J. H. van Es, et al. (2007). "Identification of stem cells in small intestine and colon by marker gene Lgr5." Nature 449(7165): 1003-1007.

Barrallo-Gimeno, A. and M. A. Nieto (2005). "The Snail genes as inducers of cell movement and survival: implications in development and cancer." Development 132(14): 3151-3161.

Barroca, V., B. Lassalle, et al. (2009). "Mouse differentiating spermatogonia can generate germinal stem cells in vivo." Nat Cell Biol 11(2): 190-196.

Basseres, D. S. and A. S. Baldwin (2006). "Nuclear factor-kappaB and inhibitor of kappaB kinase pathways in oncogenic initiation and progression." Oncogene 25(51): 6817-6830.

Batlle, E., J. T. Henderson, et al. (2002). "Beta-catenin and TCF mediate cell positioning in the intestinal epithelium by controlling the expression of EphB/ephrinB." Cell 111(2): 251-263.

Becker, C., M. C. Fantini, et al. (2006). "High resolution colonoscopy in live mice." Nat Protoc 1(6): 2900-2904.

Becker, C., M. C. Fantini, et al. (2004). "TGF-beta suppresses tumor progression in colon cancer by inhibition of IL-6 trans-signaling." Immunity 21(4): 491-501.

Bennecke, M., L. Kriegl, et al. (2010). "Ink4a/Arf and oncogene-induced senescence prevent tumor progression during alternative colorectal tumorigenesis." Cancer Cell 18(2): 135-146.

Bensaad, K., A. Tsuruta, et al. (2006). "TIGAR, a p53-inducible regulator of glycolysis and apoptosis." Cell 126(1): 107-120.

Bergers, G. and L. E. Benjamin (2003). "Tumorigenesis and the angiogenic switch." Nat Rev Cancer 3(6): 401-410.

Berx, G. and F. van Roy (2009). "Involvement of members of the cadherin superfamily in cancer." Cold Spring Harb Perspect Biol 1(6): a003129.

Bhoj, V. G. and Z. J. Chen (2009). "Ubiquitylation in innate and adaptive immunity." Nature 458(7237): 430-437.

Bilic, J., Y. L. Huang, et al. (2007). "Wnt induces LRP6 signalosomes and promotes dishevelled-dependent LRP6 phosphorylation." Science 316(5831): 1619-1622.

Bingle, L., N. J. Brown, et al. (2002). "The role of tumour-associated macrophages in tumour progression: implications for new anticancer therapies." J Pathol 196(3): 254-265.

Biswas, S., A. Chytil, et al. (2004). "Transforming growth factor beta receptor type II inactivation promotes the establishment and progression of colon cancer." Cancer Res 64(14): 4687-4692.

Blons, H. and P. Laurent-Puig (2003). "TP53 and head and neck neoplasms." Hum Mutat 21(3): 252-257.

Bollrath, J. and F. R. Greten (2009). "IKK/NF-kappaB and STAT3 pathways: central signalling hubs in inflammation-mediated tumour promotion and metastasis." EMBO Rep 10(12): 1314-1319.

Bollrath, J., T. J. Phesse, et al. (2009). "gp130-mediated Stat3 activation in enterocytes regulates cell survival and cell-cycle progression during colitis-associated tumorigenesis." Cancer Cell 15(2): 91-102.

Bonnet, D. and J. E. Dick (1997). "Human acute myeloid leukemia is organized as a hierarchy that originates from a primitive hematopoietic cell." Nat Med 3(7): 730-737.

Booth, D., J. D. Haley, et al. (2000). "Transforming growth factor-B3 protects murine small intestinal crypt stem cells and animal survival after irradiation, possibly by reducing stem-cell cycling." Int J Cancer 86(1): 53-59.

Bos, J. L., E. R. Fearon, et al. (1987). "Prevalence of ras gene mutations in human colorectal cancers." Nature 327(6120): 293-297.

Brabletz, T., A. Jung, et al. (2001). "Variable beta-catenin expression in colorectal cancers indicates tumor progression driven by the tumor environment." Proc Natl Acad Sci U S A 98(18): 10356-10361.

Brabletz, T., A. Jung, et al. (2005). "Opinion: migrating cancer stem cells - an integrated concept of malignant tumour progression." Nat Rev Cancer 5(9): 744-749.

Braunstein, S., S. C. Formenti, et al. (2008). "Acquisition of stable inducible up-regulation of nuclear factor-kappaB by tumor necrosis factor exposure confers increased radiation resistance without increased transformation in breast cancer cells." Mol Cancer Res 6(1): 78-88.

Brose, M. S., P. Volpe, et al. (2002). "BRAF and RAS mutations in human lung cancer and melanoma." Cancer Res 62(23): 6997-7000.

Castellone, M. D., H. Teramoto, et al. (2005). "Prostaglandin E2 promotes colon cancer cell growth through a Gs-axin-beta-catenin signaling axis." Science 310(5753): 1504-1510.

Cavallaro, U. and G. Christofori (2004). "Cell adhesion and signalling by cadherins and Ig-CAMs in cancer." Nat Rev Cancer 4(2): 118-132.

Ceradini, D. J., A. R. Kulkarni, et al. (2004). "Progenitor cell trafficking is regulated by hypoxic gradients through HIF-1 induction of SDF-1." Nat Med 10(8): 858-864.

Chaffer, C. L., I. Brueckmann, et al. (2011). "Normal and neoplastic nonstem cells can spontaneously convert to a stem-like state." Proc Natl Acad Sci U S A 108(19): 7950-7955.

Chan, A. T., N. Arber, et al. (2012). "Aspirin in the chemoprevention of colorectal neoplasia: an overview." Cancer Prev Res (Phila) 5(2): 164-178.

Chan, A. T., S. Ogino, et al. (2007). "Aspirin and the risk of colorectal cancer in relation to the expression of COX-2." N Engl J Med 356(21): 2131-2142.

Chan, A. T., S. Ogino, et al. (2009). "Aspirin use and survival after diagnosis of colorectal cancer." JAMA 302(6): 649-658.

Chen, J., Y. Li, et al. (2012). "A restricted cell population propagates glioblastoma growth after chemotherapy." Nature 488(7412): 522-526.

Chen, L. W., L. Egan, et al. (2003). "The two faces of IKK and NF-kappaB inhibition: prevention of systemic inflammation but increased local injury following intestinal ischemia-reperfusion." Nat Med 9(5): 575-581.

Chen, Z. J. and L. J. Sun (2009). "Nonproteolytic functions of ubiquitin in cell signaling." Mol Cell 33(3): 275-286.

Cheng, H. and C. P. Leblond (1974). "Origin, differentiation and renewal of the four main epithelial cell types in the mouse small intestine. V. Unitarian Theory of the origin of the four epithelial cell types." Am J Anat 141(4): 537-561.

Cho, R. W. and M. F. Clarke (2008). "Recent advances in cancer stem cells." Curr Opin Genet Dev 18(1): 48-53.

Christophorou, M. A., I. Ringshausen, et al. (2006). "The pathological response to DNA damage does not contribute to p53-mediated tumour suppression." Nature 443(7108): 214-217.

Clausen, B. E., C. Burkhardt, et al. (1999). "Conditional gene targeting in macrophages and granulocytes using LysMcre mice." Transgenic Res 8(4): 265-277.

Colombo, M. P. and S. Piconese (2009). "Polyps wrap mast cells and Treg within tumorigenic tentacles." Cancer Res 69(14): 5619-5622.

Crighton, D., S. Wilkinson, et al. (2006). "DRAM, a p53-induced modulator of autophagy, is critical for apoptosis." Cell 126(1): 121-134.

de Visser, K. E., A. Eichten, et al. (2006). "Paradoxical roles of the immune system during cancer development." Nat Rev Cancer 6(1): 24-37.

DeBerardinis, R. J., J. J. Lum, et al. (2008). "The biology of cancer: metabolic reprogramming fuels cell growth and proliferation." Cell Metab 7(1): 11-20.

DeLeo, A. B., G. Jay, et al. (1979). "Detection of a transformation-related antigen in chemically induced sarcomas and other transformed cells of the mouse." Proc Natl Acad Sci U S A 76(5): 2420-2424.

Delhase, M., M. Hayakawa, et al. (1999). "Positive and negative regulation of IkappaB kinase activity through IKKbeta subunit phosphorylation." Science 284(5412): 309-313.

DeNardo, D. G., P. Andreu, et al. (2010). "Interactions between lymphocytes and myeloid cells regulate pro- versus anti-tumor immunity." Cancer Metastasis Rev 29(2): 309-316.

DeNardo, D. G., J. B. Barreto, et al. (2009). "CD4(+) T cells regulate pulmonary metastasis of mammary carcinomas by enhancing protumor properties of macrophages." Cancer Cell 16(2): 91-102.

Deng, J., S. A. Miller, et al. (2002). "beta-catenin interacts with and inhibits NF-kappa B in human colon and breast cancer." Cancer Cell 2(4): 323-334.

Dittmer, D., S. Pati, et al. (1993). "Gain of function mutations in p53." Nat Genet 4(1): 42-46.

Driessens, G., B. Beck, et al. (2012). "Defining the mode of tumour growth by clonal analysis." Nature 488(7412): 527-530.

Duffy, A. and S. Kummar (2009). "Targeting mitogen-activated protein kinase kinase (MEK) in solid tumors." Target Oncol 4(4): 267-273.

Dvorak, H. F. (1986). "Tumors: wounds that do not heal. Similarities between tumor stroma generation and wound healing." N Engl J Med 315(26): 1650-1659.

Eaden, J. A., K. R. Abrams, et al. (2001). "The risk of colorectal cancer in ulcerative colitis: a meta-analysis." Gut 48(4): 526-535.

Egan, L. J., L. Eckmann, et al. (2004). "IkappaB-kinasebeta-dependent NF-kappaB activation provides radioprotection to the intestinal epithelium." Proc Natl Acad Sci U S A 101(8): 2452-2457.

Egeblad, M., E. S. Nakasone, et al. (2010). "Tumors as organs: complex tissues that interface with the entire organism." Dev Cell 18(6): 884-901.

el Marjou, F., K. P. Janssen, et al. (2004). "Tissue-specific and inducible Cre-mediated recombination in the gut epithelium." Genesis 39(3): 186-193.

Ellis, L. M. and I. J. Fidler (2010). "Finding the tumor copycat. Therapy fails, patients don't." Nat Med 16(9): 974-975.

Elyada, E., A. Pribluda, et al. (2011). "CKIalpha ablation highlights a critical role for p53 in invasiveness control." Nature 470(7334): 409-413.

Erdman, S. E., T. Poutahidis, et al. (2003). "CD4+ CD25+ regulatory T lymphocytes inhibit microbially induced colon cancer in Rag2-deficient mice." Am J Pathol 162(2): 691-702.

Erdman, S. E., V. P. Rao, et al. (2003). "CD4(+)CD25(+) regulatory lymphocytes require interleukin 10 to interrupt colon carcinogenesis in mice." Cancer Res 63(18): 6042-6050.

Erdman, S. E., J. J. Sohn, et al. (2005). "CD4+CD25+ regulatory lymphocytes induce regression of intestinal tumors in ApcMin/+ mice." Cancer Res 65(10): 3998-4004.

Estrov, Z., S. Shishodia, et al. (2003). "Resveratrol blocks interleukin-1beta-induced activation of the nuclear transcription factor NF-kappaB, inhibits proliferation, causes S-phase arrest, and induces apoptosis of acute myeloid leukemia cells." Blood 102(3): 987-995.

Fan, S., M. Gao, et al. (2005). "Role of NF-kappaB signaling in hepatocyte growth factor/scatter factor-mediated cell protection." Oncogene 24(10): 1749-1766.

Fang, Q., S. Kanugula, et al. (2005). "Function of domains of human O6-alkylguanine-DNA alkyltransferase." Biochemistry 44(46): 15396-15405.

Fearon, E. R. and B. Vogelstein (1990). "A genetic model for colorectal tumorigenesis." Cell 61(5): 759-767.

Fevr, T., S. Robine, et al. (2007). "Wnt/beta-catenin is essential for intestinal homeostasis and maintenance of intestinal stem cells." Mol Cell Biol 27(21): 7551-7559.

Fidler, I. J. and M. L. Kripke (2003). "Genomic analysis of primary tumors does not address the prevalence of metastatic cells in the population." Nat Genet 34(1): 23; author reply 25.

Fodde, R., R. Smits, et al. (2001). "APC, signal transduction and genetic instability in colorectal cancer." Nat Rev Cancer 1(1): 55-67.

Forrester, K., C. Almoguera, et al. (1987). "Detection of high incidence of K-ras oncogenes during human colon tumorigenesis." Nature 327(6120): 298-303.

Foulds, L. (1954). "The experimental study of tumor progression: a review." Cancer Res 14(5): 327-339.

Furuyama, K., Y. Kawaguchi, et al. (2011). "Continuous cell supply from a Sox9-expressing progenitor zone in adult liver, exocrine pancreas and intestine." Nat Genet 43(1): 34-41.

Galon, J., A. Costes, et al. (2006). "Type, density, and location of immune cells within human colorectal tumors predict clinical outcome." Science 313(5795): 1960-1964.

Gerbe, F., B. Brulin, et al. (2009). "DCAMKL-1 expression identifies Tuft cells rather than stem cells in the adult mouse intestinal epithelium." Gastroenterology 137(6): 2179-2180; author reply 2180-2171.

Gerbe, F., J. H. van Es, et al. (2011). "Distinct ATOH1 and Neurog3 requirements define tuft cells as a new secretory cell type in the intestinal epithelium." J Cell Biol 192(5): 767-780.

Ghosh, S. and M. Karin (2002). "Missing pieces in the NF-kappaB puzzle." Cell 109 Suppl: S81-96.

Gilbert, S. F. (2010). Developmental Biology.

Gilbertson, R. J. and J. N. Rich (2007). "Making a tumour's bed: glioblastoma stem cells and the vascular niche." Nat Rev Cancer 7(10): 733-736.

Giri, D. K. and B. B. Aggarwal (1998). "Constitutive activation of NF-kappaB causes resistance to apoptosis in human cutaneous T cell lymphoma HuT-78 cells. Autocrine role of tumor necrosis factor and reactive oxygen intermediates." J Biol Chem 273(22): 14008-14014.

Golubovskaya, V. M. and W. G. Cance (2011). "FAK and p53 Protein Interactions." Anticancer Agents Med Chem 11(7): 617-619.

Gounaris, E., N. R. Blatner, et al. (2009). "T-regulatory cells shift from a protective anti-inflammatory to a cancer-promoting proinflammatory phenotype in polyposis." Cancer Res 69(13): 5490-5497.

Gregorieff, A. and H. Clevers (2005). "Wnt signaling in the intestinal epithelium: from endoderm to cancer." Genes Dev 19(8): 877-890.

Greten, F. R., L. Eckmann, et al. (2004). "IKKbeta links inflammation and tumorigenesis in a mouse model of colitis-associated cancer." Cell 118(3): 285-296.

Grivennikov, S., E. Karin, et al. (2009). "IL-6 and Stat3 are required for survival of intestinal epithelial cells and development of colitis-associated cancer." Cancer Cell 15(2): 103-113.

Grivennikov, S. I., F. R. Greten, et al. (2010). "Immunity, inflammation, and cancer." Cell 140(6): 883-899.

Grivennikov, S. I. and M. Karin (2010). "Dangerous liaisons: STAT3 and NF-kappaB collaboration and crosstalk in cancer." Cytokine Growth Factor Rev 21(1): 11-19.

Groden, J., A. Thliveris, et al. (1991). "Identification and characterization of the familial adenomatous polyposis coli gene." Cell 66(3): 589-600.

GuhaThakurta, D. (2006). "Computational identification of transcriptional regulatory elements in DNA sequence." Nucleic Acids Res 34(12): 3585-3598.

Guo, W. and F. G. Giancotti (2004). "Integrin signalling during tumour progression." Nat Rev Mol Cell Biol 5(10): 816-826.

Guo, W., Z. Keckesova, et al. (2012). "Slug and Sox9 cooperatively determine the mammary stem cell state." Cell 148(5): 1015-1028.

Gupta, P. B., C. L. Chaffer, et al. (2009). "Cancer stem cells: mirage or reality?" Nat Med 15(9): 1010-1012.

Gupta, P. B., C. M. Fillmore, et al. (2011). "Stochastic state transitions give rise to phenotypic equilibrium in populations of cancer cells." Cell 146(4): 633-644.

Gupta, R. B., N. Harpaz, et al. (2007). "Histologic inflammation is a risk factor for progression to colorectal neoplasia in ulcerative colitis: a cohort study." Gastroenterology 133(4): 1099-1105; quiz 1340-1091.

Haigis, K. M., K. R. Kendall, et al. (2008). "Differential effects of oncogenic K-Ras and N-Ras on proliferation, differentiation and tumor progression in the colon." Nat Genet 40(5): 600-608.

Hanahan, D. and R. A. Weinberg (2000). "The hallmarks of cancer." Cell 100(1): 57-70.

Hanahan, D. and R. A. Weinberg (2011). "Hallmarks of cancer: the next generation." Cell 144(5): 646-674.

Harada, N., Y. Tamai, et al. (1999). "Intestinal polyposis in mice with a dominant stable mutation of the beta-catenin gene." EMBO J 18(21): 5931-5942.

Hlubek, F., T. Brabletz, et al. (2007). "Heterogeneous expression of Wnt/beta-catenin target genes within colorectal cancer." Int J Cancer 121(9): 1941-1948.

Hoeflich, K. P., J. Luo, et al. (2000). "Requirement for glycogen synthase kinase-3beta in cell survival and NF-kappaB activation." Nature 406(6791): 86-90.

Horst, D., J. Budczies, et al. (2009). "Invasion associated up-regulation of nuclear factor kappaB target genes in colorectal cancer." Cancer 115(21): 4946-4958.

Huang, E. H. and M. S. Wicha (2008). "Colon cancer stem cells: implications for prevention and therapy." Trends Mol Med 14(11): 503-509.

Hung, K. E., M. A. Maricevich, et al. (2010). "Development of a mouse model for sporadic and metastatic colon tumors and its use in assessing drug treatment." Proc Natl Acad Sci U S A 107(4): 1565-1570.

Hunter, K. D., E. K. Parkinson, et al. (2005). "Profiling early head and neck cancer." Nat Rev Cancer 5(2): 127-135.

Iacopetta, B. (2003). "TP53 mutation in colorectal cancer." Hum Mutat 21(3): 271-276.

Ignatiadis, M., F. Rothe, et al. (2011). "HER2-positive circulating tumor cells in breast cancer." PLoS One 6(1): e15624.

Iliopoulos, D., H. A. Hirsch, et al. (2009). "An epigenetic switch involving NF-kappaB, Lin28, Let-7 MicroRNA, and IL6 links inflammation to cell transformation." Cell 139(4): 693-706.

Iliopoulos, D., H. A. Hirsch, et al. (2011). "Inducible formation of breast cancer stem cells and their dynamic equilibrium with non-stem cancer cells via IL6 secretion." Proc Natl Acad Sci U S A 108(4): 1397-1402.

Inaba, Y., T. Ashida, et al. (2010). "Expression of the antimicrobial peptide alpha-defensin/cryptdins in intestinal crypts decreases at the initial phase of intestinal inflammation in a model of

inflammatory bowel disease, IL-10-deficient mice." Inflamm Bowel Dis 16(9): 1488-1495.
Itzkovitz, S., I. C. Blat, et al. (2012). "Optimality in the development of intestinal crypts." Cell 148(3): 608-619.
Itzkowitz, S. H. and N. Harpaz (2004). "Diagnosis and management of dysplasia in patients with inflammatory bowel diseases." Gastroenterology 126(6): 1634-1648.
Iwawaki, T., R. Akai, et al. (2004). "A transgenic mouse model for monitoring endoplasmic reticulum stress." Nat Med 10(1): 98-102.
Jackson, E. L., N. Willis, et al. (2001). "Analysis of lung tumor initiation and progression using conditional expression of oncogenic K-ras." Genes Dev 15(24): 3243-3248.
Jackson-Bernitsas, D. G., H. Ichikawa, et al. (2007). "Evidence that TNF-TNFR1-TRADD-TRAF2-RIP-TAK1-IKK pathway mediates constitutive NF-kappaB activation and proliferation in human head and neck squamous cell carcinoma." Oncogene 26(10): 1385-1397.
Jang, K. T., S. W. Chae, et al. (2002). "Coexpression of MUC1 with p53 or MUC2 correlates with lymph node metastasis in colorectal carcinomas." J Korean Med Sci 17(1): 29-33.
Janssen, K. P., P. Alberici, et al. (2006). "APC and oncogenic KRAS are synergistic in enhancing Wnt signaling in intestinal tumor formation and progression." Gastroenterology 131(4): 1096-1109.
Jemal, A., R. Siegel, et al. (2009). "Cancer statistics, 2009." CA Cancer J Clin 59(4): 225-249.
Johansson, M., D. G. Denardo, et al. (2008). "Polarized immune responses differentially regulate cancer development." Immunol Rev 222: 145-154.
Jonkers, J., R. Meuwissen, et al. (2001). "Synergistic tumor suppressor activity of BRCA2 and p53 in a conditional mouse model for breast cancer." Nat Genet 29(4): 418-425.
Joyce, J. A. and J. W. Pollard (2009). "Microenvironmental regulation of metastasis." Nat Rev Cancer 9(4): 239-252.
Junttila, M. R. and G. I. Evan (2009). "p53--a Jack of all trades but master of none." Nat Rev Cancer 9(11): 821-829.
Kaler, P., L. Augenlicht, et al. (2009). "Macrophage-derived IL-1beta stimulates Wnt signaling and growth of colon cancer cells: a crosstalk interrupted by vitamin D3." Oncogene 28(44): 3892-3902.
Kaler, P., B. N. Godasi, et al. (2009). "The NF-kappaB/AKT-dependent Induction of Wnt Signaling in Colon Cancer Cells by Macrophages and IL-1beta." Cancer Microenviron.
Kalluri, R. and M. Zeisberg (2006). "Fibroblasts in cancer." Nat Rev Cancer 6(5): 392-401.

Karin, M. (2006). "Nuclear factor-kappaB in cancer development and progression." Nature 441(7092): 431-436.

Karin, M., Y. Cao, et al. (2002). "NF-kappaB in cancer: from innocent bystander to major culprit." Nat Rev Cancer 2(4): 301-310.

Karnoub, A. E., A. B. Dash, et al. (2007). "Mesenchymal stem cells within tumour stroma promote breast cancer metastasis." Nature 449(7162): 557-563.

Kato, S., S. Y. Han, et al. (2003). "Understanding the function-structure and function-mutation relationships of p53 tumor suppressor protein by high-resolution missense mutation analysis." Proc Natl Acad Sci U S A 100(14): 8424-8429.

Kawauchi, K., K. Araki, et al. (2008). "p53 regulates glucose metabolism through an IKK-NF-kappaB pathway and inhibits cell transformation." Nat Cell Biol 10(5): 611-618.

Kazanskaya, O., A. Glinka, et al. (2004). "R-Spondin2 is a secreted activator of Wnt/beta-catenin signaling and is required for Xenopus myogenesis." Dev Cell 7(4): 525-534.

Kessenbrock, K., V. Plaks, et al. (2010). "Matrix metalloproteinases: regulators of the tumor microenvironment." Cell 141(1): 52-67.

Kim, K. A., M. Kakitani, et al. (2005). "Mitogenic influence of human R-spondin1 on the intestinal epithelium." Science 309(5738): 1256-1259.

Kimelman, D. and W. Xu (2006). "beta-catenin destruction complex: insights and questions from a structural perspective." Oncogene 25(57): 7482-7491.

Kinzler, K. W., M. C. Nilbert, et al. (1991). "Identification of FAP locus genes from chromosome 5q21." Science 253(5020): 661-665.

Kinzler, K. W. and B. Vogelstein (1996). "Lessons from hereditary colorectal cancer." Cell 87(2): 159-170.

Klaus, A. and W. Birchmeier (2008). "Wnt signalling and its impact on development and cancer." Nat Rev Cancer 8(5): 387-398.

Klymkowsky, M. W. and P. Savagner (2009). "Epithelial-mesenchymal transition: a cancer researcher's conceptual friend and foe." Am J Pathol 174(5): 1588-1593.

Kohrt, H. E., N. Nouri, et al. (2005). "Profile of immune cells in axillary lymph nodes predicts disease-free survival in breast cancer." PLoS Med 2(9): e284.

Korinek, V., N. Barker, et al. (1998). "Depletion of epithelial stem-cell compartments in the small intestine of mice lacking Tcf-4." Nat Genet 19(4): 379-383.

Korinek, V., N. Barker, et al. (1997). "Constitutive transcriptional activation by a beta-catenin-Tcf complex in APC-/- colon carcinoma." Science 275(5307): 1784-1787.

Kortylewski, M., H. Xin, et al. (2009). "Regulation of the IL-23 and IL-12 balance by Stat3 signaling in the tumor microenvironment." Cancer Cell 15(2): 114-123.
Koumakpayi, I. H., C. Le Page, et al. (2010). "Hierarchical clustering of immunohistochemical analysis of the activated ErbB/PI3K/Akt/NF-kappaB signalling pathway and prognostic significance in prostate cancer." Br J Cancer 102(7): 1163-1173.
Kujawski, M., M. Kortylewski, et al. (2008). "Stat3 mediates myeloid cell-dependent tumor angiogenesis in mice." J Clin Invest 118(10): 3367-3377.
Kusaba, T., T. Nakayama, et al. (2005). "Expression of p-STAT3 in human colorectal adenocarcinoma and adenoma; correlation with clinicopathological factors." J Clin Pathol 58(8): 833-838.
Laghi, L., P. Bianchi, et al. (2009). "CD3+ cells at the invasive margin of deeply invading (pT3-T4) colorectal cancer and risk of post-surgical metastasis: a longitudinal study." Lancet Oncol 10(9): 877-884.
Lander, E. S., L. M. Linton, et al. (2001). "Initial sequencing and analysis of the human genome." Nature 409(6822): 860-921.
Lane, D. P. (1992). "Cancer. p53, guardian of the genome." Nature 358(6381): 15-16.
Langowski, J. L., R. A. Kastelein, et al. (2007). "Swords into plowshares: IL-23 repurposes tumor immune surveillance." Trends Immunol 28(5): 207-212.
Langowski, J. L., X. Zhang, et al. (2006). "IL-23 promotes tumour incidence and growth." Nature 442(7101): 461-465.
Le Page, C., I. H. Koumakpayi, et al. (2005). "EGFR and Her-2 regulate the constitutive activation of NF-kappaB in PC-3 prostate cancer cells." Prostate 65(2): 130-140.
Levine, A. J. (1997). "p53, the cellular gatekeeper for growth and division." Cell 88(3): 323-331.
Levine, A. J., W. Hu, et al. (2006). "The P53 pathway: what questions remain to be explored?" Cell Death Differ 13(6): 1027-1036.
Lin, W. W. and M. Karin (2007). "A cytokine-mediated link between innate immunity, inflammation, and cancer." J Clin Invest 117(5): 1175-1183.
Ling, J., Y. Kang, et al. (2012). "KrasG12D-induced IKK2/beta/NF-kappaB activation by IL-1alpha and p62 feedforward loops is required for development of pancreatic ductal adenocarcinoma." Cancer Cell 21(1): 105-120.
Liou, H. C., M. R. Boothby, et al. (1990). "A new member of the leucine zipper class of proteins that binds to the HLA DR alpha promoter." Science 247(4950): 1581-1584.

Lobo, N. A., Y. Shimono, et al. (2007). "The biology of cancer stem cells." Annu Rev Cell Dev Biol 23: 675-699.

Lopez-Garcia, C., A. M. Klein, et al. (2010). "Intestinal stem cell replacement follows a pattern of neutral drift." Science 330(6005): 822-825.

Lu, S. L., H. Herrington, et al. (2006). "Loss of transforming growth factor-beta type II receptor promotes metastatic head-and-neck squamous cell carcinoma." Genes Dev 20(10): 1331-1342.

Luche, H., O. Weber, et al. (2007). "Faithful activation of an extra-bright red fluorescent protein in "knock-in" Cre-reporter mice ideally suited for lineage tracing studies." Eur J Immunol 37(1): 43-53.

Luo, F., D. G. Brooks, et al. (2009). "Mutated K-ras(Asp12) promotes tumourigenesis in Apc(Min) mice more in the large than the small intestines, with synergistic effects between K-ras and Wnt pathways." Int J Exp Pathol 90(5): 558-574.

Madison, B. B., L. Dunbar, et al. (2002). "Cis elements of the villin gene control expression in restricted domains of the vertical (crypt) and horizontal (duodenum, cecum) axes of the intestine." J Biol Chem 277(36): 33275-33283.

Malkin, D., F. P. Li, et al. (1990). "Germ line p53 mutations in a familial syndrome of breast cancer, sarcomas, and other neoplasms." Science 250(4985): 1233-1238.

Mani, S. A., W. Guo, et al. (2008). "The epithelial-mesenchymal transition generates cells with properties of stem cells." Cell 133(4): 704-715.

Mantovani, A. (2010). "Molecular pathways linking inflammation and cancer." Curr Mol Med 10(4): 369-373.

Mantovani, A., P. Allavena, et al. (2008). "Cancer-related inflammation." Nature 454(7203): 436-444.

Mantovani, A., S. Sozzani, et al. (2002). "Macrophage polarization: tumor-associated macrophages as a paradigm for polarized M2 mononuclear phagocytes." Trends Immunol 23(11): 549-555.

Marsh, V., D. J. Winton, et al. (2008). "Epithelial Pten is dispensable for intestinal homeostasis but suppresses adenoma development and progression after Apc mutation." Nat Genet 40(12): 1436-1444.

Marshman, E., C. Booth, et al. (2002). "The intestinal epithelial stem cell." Bioessays 24(1): 91-98.

Matoba, S., J. G. Kang, et al. (2006). "p53 regulates mitochondrial respiration." Science 312(5780): 1650-1653.

Medema, J. P. and L. Vermeulen (2011). "Microenvironmental regulation of stem cells in intestinal homeostasis and cancer." Nature 474(7351): 318-326.

Meek, D. W. (2009). "Tumour suppression by p53: a role for the DNA damage response?" Nat Rev Cancer 9(10): 714-723.

Meining, A., E. Frimberger, et al. (2008). "Detection of cholangiocarcinoma *in vivo* using miniprobe-based confocal fluorescence microscopy." Clin Gastroenterol Hepatol 6(9): 1057-1060.

Meylan, E., A. L. Dooley, et al. (2009). "Requirement for NF-kappaB signalling in a mouse model of lung adenocarcinoma." Nature 462(7269): 104-107.

Micalizzi, D. S., S. M. Farabaugh, et al. (2010). "Epithelial-mesenchymal transition in cancer: parallels between normal development and tumor progression." J Mammary Gland Biol Neoplasia 15(2): 117-134.

Miyaki, M., M. Konishi, et al. (1994). "Characteristics of somatic mutation of the adenomatous polyposis coli gene in colorectal tumors." Cancer Res 54(11): 3011-3020.

Mohamed, M. M. and B. F. Sloane (2006). "Cysteine cathepsins: multifunctional enzymes in cancer." Nat Rev Cancer 6(10): 764-775.

Montgomery, R. K., D. L. Carlone, et al. (2011). "Mouse telomerase reverse transcriptase (mTert) expression marks slowly cycling intestinal stem cells." Proc Natl Acad Sci U S A 108(1): 179-184.

Moolenbeek, C. and E. J. Ruitenberg (1981). "The "Swiss roll": a simple technique for histological studies of the rodent intestine." Lab Anim 15(1): 57-59.

Morel, A. P., M. Lievre, et al. (2008). "Generation of breast cancer stem cells through epithelial-mesenchymal transition." PLoS One 3(8): e2888.

Morin, P. J. (1997). "Activation of beta -Catenin-Tcf Signaling in Colon Cancer by Mutations in beta -Catenin or APC." Science 275(5307): 1787-1790.

Morin, P. J., A. B. Sparks, et al. (1997). "Activation of beta-catenin-Tcf signaling in colon cancer by mutations in beta-catenin or APC." Science 275(5307): 1787-1790.

Mougiakakos, D., A. Choudhury, et al. (2010). "Regulatory T cells in cancer." Adv Cancer Res 107: 57-117.

Muller, A., B. Homey, et al. (2001). "Involvement of chemokine receptors in breast cancer metastasis." Nature 410(6824): 50-56.

Murdoch, C., M. Muthana, et al. (2008). "The role of myeloid cells in the promotion of tumour angiogenesis." Nat Rev Cancer 8(8): 618-631.

Nagashima, K., V. G. Sasseville, et al. (2006). "Rapid TNFR1-dependent lymphocyte depletion *in vivo* with a selective chemical inhibitor of IKKbeta." Blood 107(11): 4266-4273.

Najdi, R., R. F. Holcombe, et al. (2011). "Wnt signaling and colon carcinogenesis: beyond APC." J Carcinog 10: 5.

Naoki, K., T. H. Chen, et al. (2002). "Missense mutations of the BRAF gene in human lung adenocarcinoma." Cancer Res 62(23): 7001-7003.

Network, C. G. A. (2012). "Comprehensive molecular characterization of human colon and rectal cancer." Nature 487(7407): 330-337.

Nowell, P. C. (1976). "The clonal evolution of tumor cell populations." Science 194(4260): 23-28.

Nusse, R. and H. E. Varmus (1982). "Many tumors induced by the mouse mammary tumor virus contain a provirus integrated in the same region of the host genome." Cell 31(1): 99-109.

Ogata, H., A. Sekikawa, et al. (2010). "GROalpha promotes invasion of colorectal cancer cells." Oncol Rep 24(6): 1479-1486.

Oguma, K., H. Oshima, et al. (2008). "Activated macrophages promote Wnt signalling through tumour necrosis factor-alpha in gastric tumour cells." EMBO J 27(12): 1671-1681.

Ojalvo, L. S., W. King, et al. (2009). "High-density gene expression analysis of tumor-associated macrophages from mouse mammary tumors." Am J Pathol 174(3): 1048-1064.

Ojalvo, L. S., C. A. Whittaker, et al. (2010). "Gene expression analysis of macrophages that facilitate tumor invasion supports a role for Wnt-signaling in mediating their activity in primary mammary tumors." J Immunol 184(2): 702-712.

Oren, M. (2003). "Decision making by p53: life, death and cancer." Cell Death Differ 10(4): 431-442.

Oshima, H., M. Oshima, et al. (1997). "Morphological and molecular processes of polyp formation in Apc(delta716) knockout mice." Cancer Res 57(9): 1644-1649.

Oshima, M. and M. M. Taketo (2002). "COX selectivity and animal models for colon cancer." Curr Pharm Des 8(12): 1021-1034.

Ostrand-Rosenberg, S. and P. Sinha (2009). "Myeloid-derived suppressor cells: linking inflammation and cancer." J Immunol 182(8): 4499-4506.

Owen, K. A., M. Y. Abshire, et al. (2011). "FAK regulates intestinal epithelial cell survival and proliferation during mucosal wound healing." PLoS One 6(8): e23123.

Paez, J. G., P. A. Janne, et al. (2004). "EGFR mutations in lung cancer: correlation with clinical response to gefitinib therapy." Science 304(5676): 1497-1500.

Pahl, H. L. (1999). "Activators and target genes of Rel/NF-kappaB transcription factors." Oncogene 18(49): 6853-6866.
Palermo, C. and J. A. Joyce (2008). "Cysteine cathepsin proteases as pharmacological targets in cancer." Trends Pharmacol Sci 29(1): 22-28.
Pasparakis, M., L. Alexopoulou, et al. (1996). "Immune and inflammatory responses in TNF alpha-deficient mice: a critical requirement for TNF alpha in the formation of primary B cell follicles, follicular dendritic cell networks and germinal centers, and in the maturation of the humoral immune response." J Exp Med 184(4): 1397-1411.
Patel, V., H. M. Rosenfeldt, et al. (2007). "Persistent activation of Rac1 in squamous carcinomas of the head and neck: evidence for an EGFR/Vav2 signaling axis involved in cell invasion." Carcinogenesis 28(6): 1145-1152.
Peinado, H., E. Ballestar, et al. (2004). "Snail mediates E-cadherin repression by the recruitment of the Sin3A/histone deacetylase 1 (HDAC1)/HDAC2 complex." Mol Cell Biol 24(1): 306-319.
Peller, S. and V. Rotter (2003). "TP53 in hematological cancer: low incidence of mutations with significant clinical relevance." Hum Mutat 21(3): 277-284.
Perkins, N. D. (2006). "Post-translational modifications regulating the activity and function of the nuclear factor kappa B pathway." Oncogene 25(51): 6717-6730.
Perkins, N. D. (2012). "The diverse and complex roles of NF-kappaB subunits in cancer." Nat Rev Cancer 12(2): 121-132.
Perkins, N. D., N. L. Edwards, et al. (1993). "A cooperative interaction between NF-kappa B and Sp1 is required for HIV-1 enhancer activation." EMBO J 12(9): 3551-3558.
Peterson, J., S. Garges, et al. (2009). "The NIH Human Microbiome Project." Genome Res 19(12): 2317-2323.
Phelps, R. A., S. Chidester, et al. (2009). "A two-step model for colon adenoma initiation and progression caused by APC loss." Cell 137(4): 623-634.
Pianetti, S., M. Arsura, et al. (2001). "Her-2/neu overexpression induces NF-kappaB via a PI3-kinase/Akt pathway involving calpain-mediated degradation of IkappaB-alpha that can be inhibited by the tumor suppressor PTEN." Oncogene 20(11): 1287-1299.
Pikarsky, E., R. M. Porat, et al. (2004). "NF-kappaB functions as a tumour promoter in inflammation-associated cancer." Nature 431(7007): 461-466.
Pinto, D. and H. Clevers (2005). "Wnt, stem cells and cancer in the intestine." Biol Cell 97(3): 185-196.

Pohl, H., T. Rosch, et al. (2008). "Miniprobe confocal laser microscopy for the detection of invisible neoplasia in patients with Barrett's oesophagus." Gut 57(12): 1648-1653.

Polakis, P. (1999). "The oncogenic activation of beta-catenin." Curr Opin Genet Dev 9(1): 15-21.

Pollard, J. W. (2004). "Tumour-educated macrophages promote tumour progression and metastasis." Nat Rev Cancer 4(1): 71-78.

Polyak, K. and R. A. Weinberg (2009). "Transitions between epithelial and mesenchymal states: acquisition of malignant and stem cell traits." Nat Rev Cancer 9(4): 265-273.

Popivanova, B. K., K. Kitamura, et al. (2008). "Blocking TNF-alpha in mice reduces colorectal carcinogenesis associated with chronic colitis." J Clin Invest 118(2): 560-570.

Potten, C. S., C. Booth, et al. (1997). "The intestinal epithelial stem cell: the mucosal governor." Int J Exp Pathol 78(4): 219-243.

Potten, C. S., C. Booth, et al. (2003). "Identification of a putative intestinal stem cell and early lineage marker; musashi-1." Differentiation 71(1): 28-41.

Prasad, S., J. Ravindran, et al. (2010). "NF-kappaB and cancer: how intimate is this relationship." Mol Cell Biochem 336(1-2): 25-37.

Preston, S. L., W. M. Wong, et al. (2003). "Bottom-up histogenesis of colorectal adenomas: origin in the monocryptal adenoma and initial expansion by crypt fission." Cancer Res 63(13): 3819-3825.

Purandare, S., K. Offenbartl, et al. (1989). "Increased gut permeability to fluorescein isothiocyanate-dextran after total parenteral nutrition in the rat." Scand J Gastroenterol 24(6): 678-682.

Qian, B. Z. and J. W. Pollard (2010). "Macrophage diversity enhances tumor progression and metastasis." Cell 141(1): 39-51.

Quante, M. and T. C. Wang (2009). "Stem cells in gastroenterology and hepatology." Nat Rev Gastroenterol Hepatol 6(12): 724-737.

Reya, T., S. J. Morrison, et al. (2001). "Stem cells, cancer, and cancer stem cells." Nature 414(6859): 105-111.

Rius, J., M. Guma, et al. (2008). "NF-kappaB links innate immunity to the hypoxic response through transcriptional regulation of HIF-1alpha." Nature 453(7196): 807-811.

Rizk, P. and N. Barker (2012). "Gut stem cells in tissue renewal and disease: methods, markers, and myths." Wiley Interdiscip Rev Syst Biol Med 4(5): 475-496.

Rosen, J. M. and C. T. Jordan (2009). "The increasing complexity of the cancer stem cell paradigm." Science 324(5935): 1670-1673.

Rothwell, P. M., F. G. Fowkes, et al. (2011). "Effect of daily aspirin on long-term risk of death due to cancer: analysis of individual patient data from randomised trials." Lancet 377(9759): 31-41.

Rupec, R. A., F. Jundt, et al. (2005). "Stroma-mediated dysregulation of myelopoiesis in mice lacking I kappa B alpha." Immunity 22(4): 479-491.

Rupec, R. A., D. Poujol, et al. (1999). "Structural analysis, expression, and chromosomal localization of the mouse ikba gene." Immunogenetics 49(5): 395-403.

Rutter, M., B. Saunders, et al. (2004). "Severity of inflammation is a risk factor for colorectal neoplasia in ulcerative colitis." Gastroenterology 126(2): 451-459.

Sablina, A. A., A. V. Budanov, et al. (2005). "The antioxidant function of the p53 tumor suppressor." Nat Med 11(12): 1306-1313.

Sakaguchi, S. (2005). "Naturally arising Foxp3-expressing CD25+CD4+ regulatory T cells in immunological tolerance to self and non-self." Nat Immunol 6(4): 345-352.

Sanchez-Cespedes, M., P. Parrella, et al. (2002). "Inactivation of LKB1/STK11 is a common event in adenocarcinomas of the lung." Cancer Res 62(13): 3659-3662.

Sanger, N., K. E. Effenberger, et al. (2011). "Disseminated tumor cells in the bone marrow of patients with ductal carcinoma in situ." Int J Cancer 129(10): 2522-2526.

Sangiorgi, E. and M. R. Capecchi (2008). "Bmi1 is expressed *in vivo* in intestinal stem cells." Nat Genet 40(7): 915-920.

Sangiorgi, E. and M. R. Capecchi (2009). "Bmi1 lineage tracing identifies a self-renewing pancreatic acinar cell subpopulation capable of maintaining pancreatic organ homeostasis." Proc Natl Acad Sci U S A 106(17): 7101-7106.

Sansom, O. J., V. Meniel, et al. (2006). "Loss of Apc allows phenotypic manifestation of the transforming properties of an endogenous K-ras oncogene *in vivo*." Proc Natl Acad Sci U S A 103(38): 14122-14127.

Sansom, O. J., K. R. Reed, et al. (2004). "Loss of Apc *in vivo* immediately perturbs Wnt signaling, differentiation, and migration." Genes Dev 18(12): 1385-1390.

Sato, T., J. H. van Es, et al. (2011). "Paneth cells constitute the niche for Lgr5 stem cells in intestinal crypts." Nature 469(7330): 415-418.

Sato, T., R. G. Vries, et al. (2009). "Single Lgr5 stem cells build crypt-villus structures *in vitro* without a mesenchymal niche." Nature 459(7244): 262-265.

Scheel, C., E. N. Eaton, et al. (2011). "Paracrine and autocrine signals induce and maintain mesenchymal and stem cell states in the breast." Cell 145(6): 926-940.

Scheidereit, C. (2006). "IkappaB kinase complexes: gateways to NF-kappaB activation and transcription." Oncogene 25(51): 6685-6705.

Schepers, A. G., H. J. Snippert, et al. (2012). "Lineage tracing reveals Lgr5+ stem cell activity in mouse intestinal adenomas." Science 337(6095): 730-735.

Schioppa, T., B. Uranchimeg, et al. (2003). "Regulation of the chemokine receptor CXCR4 by hypoxia." J Exp Med 198(9): 1391-1402.

Schmalhofer, O., S. Brabletz, et al. (2009). "E-cadherin, beta-catenin, and ZEB1 in malignant progression of cancer." Cancer Metastasis Rev 28(1-2): 151-166.

Schuijer, M. and E. M. Berns (2003). "TP53 and ovarian cancer." Hum Mutat 21(3): 285-291.

Schwerbrock, N. M., M. K. Makkink, et al. (2004). "Interleukin 10-deficient mice exhibit defective colonic Muc2 synthesis before and after induction of colitis by commensal bacteria." Inflamm Bowel Dis 10(6): 811-823.

Scian, M. J., K. E. Stagliano, et al. (2005). "Tumor-derived p53 mutants induce NF-kappaB2 gene expression." Mol Cell Biol 25(22): 10097-10110.

Scortegagna, M., C. Cataisson, et al. (2008). "HIF-1alpha regulates epithelial inflammation by cell autonomous NFkappaB activation and paracrine stromal remodeling." Blood 111(7): 3343-3354.

Sen, R. and D. Baltimore (1986). "Multiple nuclear factors interact with the immunoglobulin enhancer sequences." Cell 46(5): 705-716.

Senftleben, U., Y. Cao, et al. (2001). "Activation by IKKalpha of a second, evolutionary conserved, NF-kappa B signaling pathway." Science 293(5534): 1495-1499.

Sethi, G., K. S. Ahn, et al. (2007). "Epidermal growth factor (EGF) activates nuclear factor-kappaB through IkappaBalpha kinase-independent but EGF receptor-kinase dependent tyrosine 42 phosphorylation of IkappaBalpha." Oncogene 26(52): 7324-7332.

Shaulsky, G., N. Goldfinger, et al. (1991). "Alterations in tumor development *in vivo* mediated by expression of wild type or mutant p53 proteins." Cancer Res 51(19): 5232-5237.

Shibata, H., K. Toyama, et al. (1997). "Rapid colorectal adenoma formation initiated by conditional targeting of the Apc gene." Science 278(5335): 120-123.

Shih, I. M., T. L. Wang, et al. (2001). "Top-down morphogenesis of colorectal tumors." Proc Natl Acad Sci U S A 98(5): 2640-2645.

Sica, A., A. Saccani, et al. (2000). "Autocrine production of IL-10 mediates defective IL-12 production and NF-kappa B activation in tumor-associated macrophages." J Immunol 164(2): 762-767.

Simons, B. D. and H. Clevers (2011). "Strategies for homeostatic stem cell self-renewal in adult tissues." Cell 145(6): 851-862.

Singh, A. and J. Settleman (2010). "EMT, cancer stem cells and drug resistance: an emerging axis of evil in the war on cancer." Oncogene 29(34): 4741-4751.

Smyth, M. J., G. P. Dunn, et al. (2006). "Cancer immunosurveillance and immunoediting: the roles of immunity in suppressing tumor development and shaping tumor immunogenicity." Adv Immunol 90: 1-50.

Smyth, M. J., M. W. Teng, et al. (2006). "CD4+CD25+ T regulatory cells suppress NK cell-mediated immunotherapy of cancer." J Immunol 176(3): 1582-1587.

Snippert, H. J., L. G. van der Flier, et al. (2010). "Intestinal crypt homeostasis results from neutral competition between symmetrically dividing Lgr5 stem cells." Cell 143(1): 134-144.

Soler, A. P., R. D. Miller, et al. (1999). "Increased tight junctional permeability is associated with the development of colon cancer." Carcinogenesis 20(8): 1425-1431.

Solinas, G., G. Germano, et al. (2009). "Tumor-associated macrophages (TAM) as major players of the cancer-related inflammation." J Leukoc Biol 86(5): 1065-1073.

Spiegelman, V. S., T. J. Slaga, et al. (2000). "Wnt/beta-catenin signaling induces the expression and activity of betaTrCP ubiquitin ligase receptor." Mol Cell 5(5): 877-882.

Steinbrecher, K. A., W. Wilson, 3rd, et al. (2005). "Glycogen synthase kinase 3beta functions to specify gene-specific, NF-kappaB-dependent transcription." Mol Cell Biol 25(19): 8444-8455.

Stephens, P., C. Hunter, et al. (2004). "Lung cancer: intragenic ERBB2 kinase mutations in tumours." Nature 431(7008): 525-526.

Subramanian, A., P. Tamayo, et al. (2005). "Gene set enrichment analysis: a knowledge-based approach for interpreting genome-wide expression profiles." Proc Natl Acad Sci U S A 102(43): 15545-15550.

Swann, J. B. and M. J. Smyth (2007). "Immune surveillance of tumors." J Clin Invest 117(5): 1137-1146.

Takeda, N., R. Jain, et al. (2011). "Interconversion Between Intestinal Stem Cell Populations in Distinct Niches." Science 334(6061): 1420-1424.

Taketo, M. M. and W. Edelmann (2009). "Mouse models of colon cancer." Gastroenterology 136(3): 780-798.

Talchai, C., S. Xuan, et al. (2012). "Pancreatic beta Cell Dedifferentiation as a Mechanism of Diabetic beta Cell Failure." Cell 150(6): 1223-1234.

Tenesa, A. and M. G. Dunlop (2009). "New insights into the aetiology of colorectal cancer from genome-wide association studies." Nat Rev Genet 10(6): 353-358.

Thiery, J. P., H. Acloque, et al. (2009). "Epithelial-mesenchymal transitions in development and disease." Cell 139(5): 871-890.

Thiery, J. P. and J. P. Sleeman (2006). "Complex networks orchestrate epithelial-mesenchymal transitions." Nat Rev Mol Cell Biol 7(2): 131-142.

Thomas, S. M., N. E. Bhola, et al. (2006). "Cross-talk between G protein-coupled receptor and epidermal growth factor receptor signaling pathways contributes to growth and invasion of head and neck squamous cell carcinoma." Cancer Res 66(24): 11831-11839.

Tian, H., B. Biehs, et al. (2011). "A reserve stem cell population in small intestine renders Lgr5-positive cells dispensable." Nature 478(7368): 255-259.

Umar, S., S. Sarkar, et al. (2009). "Functional cross-talk between beta-catenin and NFkappaB signaling pathways in colonic crypts of mice in response to progastrin." J Biol Chem 284(33): 22274-22284.

Uronis, J. M., M. Muhlbauer, et al. (2009). "Modulation of the intestinal microbiota alters colitis-associated colorectal cancer susceptibility." PLoS One 4(6): e6026.

Valastyan, S. and R. A. Weinberg (2011). "Tumor metastasis: molecular insights and evolving paradigms." Cell 147(2): 275-292.

Valdes-Mora, F., T. Gomez del Pulgar, et al. (2009). "TWIST1 overexpression is associated with nodal invasion and male sex in primary colorectal cancer." Ann Surg Oncol 16(1): 78-87.

Vallabhapurapu, S. and M. Karin (2009). "Regulation and function of NF-kappaB transcription factors in the immune system." Annu Rev Immunol 27: 693-733.

van de Wetering, M., E. Sancho, et al. (2002). "The beta-catenin/TCF-4 complex imposes a crypt progenitor phenotype on colorectal cancer cells." Cell 111(2): 241-250.

Van der Flier, L. G., J. Sabates-Bellver, et al. (2007). "The Intestinal Wnt/TCF Signature." Gastroenterology 132(2): 628-632.

van der Flier, L. G., M. E. van Gijn, et al. (2009). "Transcription factor achaete scute-like 2 controls intestinal stem cell fate." Cell 136(5): 903-912.

Vatsyayan, J., G. Qing, et al. (2008). "SUMO1 modification of NF-kappaB2/p100 is essential for stimuli-induced p100 phosphorylation and processing." EMBO Rep 9(9): 885-890.

Vega, K. J., R. May, et al. (2012). "Identification of the putative intestinal stem cell marker doublecortin and CaM kinase-like-1 in Barrett's esophagus and esophageal adenocarcinoma." J Gastroenterol Hepatol 27(4): 773-780.

Vermeulen, L., E. M. F. De Sousa, et al. (2010). "Wnt activity defines colon cancer stem cells and is regulated by the microenvironment." Nat Cell Biol 12(5): 468-476.

Vitale-Cross, L., P. Amornphimoltham, et al. (2004). "Conditional expression of K-ras in an epithelial compartment that includes the stem cells is sufficient to promote squamous cell carcinogenesis." Cancer Res 64(24): 8804-8807.

Waldner, M. J. and M. F. Neurath (2009). "Chemically induced mouse models of colitis." Curr Protoc Pharmacol Chapter 5: Unit 5 55.

Waldner, M. J., S. Wirtz, et al. (2011). "Confocal laser endomicroscopy and narrow-band imaging-aided endoscopy for *in vivo* imaging of colitis and colon cancer in mice." Nat Protoc 6(9): 1471-1481.

Wang, S. P., W. L. Wang, et al. (2009). "p53 controls cancer cell invasion by inducing the MDM2-mediated degradation of Slug." Nat Cell Biol 11(6): 694-704.

Wang, X., O. Tully, et al. (2011). "Epithelial tight junctional changes in colorectal cancer tissues." ScientificWorldJournal 11: 826-841.

Watanabe, T., T. Kobunai, et al. (2011). "Differential gene expression signatures between colorectal cancers with and without KRAS mutations: crosstalk between the KRAS pathway and other signalling pathways." Eur J Cancer 47(13): 1946-1954.

Webster, G. A. and N. D. Perkins (1999). "Transcriptional cross talk between NF-kappaB and p53." Mol Cell Biol 19(5): 3485-3495.

Weisz, L., A. Damalas, et al. (2007). "Mutant p53 enhances nuclear factor kappaB activation by tumor necrosis factor alpha in cancer cells." Cancer Res 67(6): 2396-2401.

Werner, S. L., D. Barken, et al. (2005). "Stimulus specificity of gene expression programs determined by temporal control of IKK activity." Science 309(5742): 1857-1861.

Winston, J. T., P. Strack, et al. (1999). "The SCFbeta-TRCP-ubiquitin ligase complex associates specifically with phosphorylated destruction motifs in IkappaBalpha and beta-catenin and stimulates IkappaBalpha ubiquitination *in vitro*." Genes Dev 13(3): 270-283.

Wolf, D., N. Harris, et al. (1984). "Reconstitution of p53 expression in a nonproducer Ab-MuLV-transformed cell line by transfection of a functional p53 gene." Cell 38(1): 119-126.

Wood, L. D., D. W. Parsons, et al. (2007). "The genomic landscapes of human breast and colorectal cancers." Science 318(5853): 1108-1113.

Wright, C. J., T. Zhuang, et al. (2009). "Hyperoxia-induced NF-kappaB activation occurs via a maturationally sensitive atypical pathway." Am J Physiol Lung Cell Mol Physiol 296(3): L296-306.

Wu, X., X. Tu, et al. (2008). "Rac1 activation controls nuclear localization of beta-catenin during canonical Wnt signaling." Cell 133(2): 340-353.

Yan, K. S., L. A. Chia, et al. (2012). "The intestinal stem cell markers Bmi1 and Lgr5 identify two functionally distinct populations." Proc Natl Acad Sci U S A 109(2): 466-471.

Yang, J. and R. A. Weinberg (2008). "Epithelial-mesenchymal transition: at the crossroads of development and tumor metastasis." Dev Cell 14(6): 818-829.

Yilmaz, M. and G. Christofori (2009). "EMT, the cytoskeleton, and cancer cell invasion." Cancer Metastasis Rev 28(1-2): 15-33.

Yin, M. J., Y. Yamamoto, et al. (1998). "The anti-inflammatory agents aspirin and salicylate inhibit the activity of I(kappa)B kinase-beta." Nature 396(6706): 77-80.

Yochum, G. S., S. McWeeney, et al. (2007). "Serial analysis of chromatin occupancy identifies beta-catenin target genes in colorectal carcinoma cells." Proc Natl Acad Sci U S A 104(9): 3324-3329.

Yoshida, H. (2007). "Unconventional splicing of XBP-1 mRNA in the unfolded protein response." Antioxid Redox Signal 9(12): 2323-2333.

Yu, H., D. Pardoll, et al. (2009). "STATs in cancer inflammation and immunity: a leading role for STAT3." Nat Rev Cancer 9(11): 798-809.

Yu, J., M. A. Vodyanik, et al. (2007). "Induced pluripotent stem cell lines derived from human somatic cells." Science 318(5858): 1917-1920.

Zhu, L., P. Gibson, et al. (2009). "Prominin 1 marks intestinal stem cells that are susceptible to neoplastic transformation." Nature 457(7229): 603-607.

Abbreviations

AOM	azoxymethane
APC	adenomatous polyposis coli
BrdU	bromodesoxyuridine
CAC	colitis associated colon cancer
CBC	crypt base comlumnar
CBP	CREB-binding protein
CCL	chemokine ligand C-C motif
CD	cluster of differentiation
CD	Crohn's disease
CK1a	casein kinase 1 alpha
CRC	colorectal cancer
CREB	cAMP response element-binding protein
CSC	cancer stem cell
CSF1	colony stimulating factor 1
CTL	cytotoxic T cells
CXCL	chemokine ligand C-X-C motif
DAPI	4',6-diamidino-2-phenylindole
DNA	deoxyribonucleic acid
dNTP	deoxynucleotide triphosphate
DSS	dextran sulphate sodium
EGF	endothelial growth factor
EMT	epithelial–mesenchymal transition
FAK	focal adhesion kinase
FAP	familial adenomatous polyposis
FCS	fetal calf serum
FGF	fibroblast growth factor
h	hour

H&E	haematoxylin & eosin
HGF	hepatocyte growth factor
HRP	horseradish peroxidase
i.p.	intra-peritoneal
i.v.	intravenous
IBD	inflammatory bowel disease
IEC	intestinal epithelial cell
IFNg	interferon gamma
IHC	immunohistochemistry
IKK	I kappa B kinase
IL	interleukin
iPSC	induced pluripotent stem cells
IκBα	nuclear factor kappa-b inhibitor
K-Ras	Kirsten-Ras
LEF	lymphoid enhancer-binding factor 1
LIF	leukemia inhibitory factor
LOH	loss of heterozygosity
MDSC	myeloid-derived suppressor cells
MHC	major histocompatibility complex
min	minute
MMP	matrix-metalloproteinase
MMTV	mouse mammary tumor virus
MyD88	myeloid differentiation primary response gene 88
NF-kB	nuclear factor kappa B
NIH	National Institutes of Health
NK	natural killer
NSAID	nonsteroidal anti-inflammatory drugs

PBS	phosphate buffered saline
PCR	polymerase chain reaction
PDAC	pancreatic ductal adenocarcinoma
PFA	paraformaldehyde
PGE2	prostaglandin E2
PP2A	protein phosphatase 2 A
Rac1	Ras-related C3 botulinum toxin substrate 1
RNA	ribonucleic acid
ROS	reactive oxygen species
sec	second
SEM	standard error of the mean
SMAD	sma- and mad-related protein 1
STAT	signal transducer and activator of transcription
TAM	tumor associated macrophages
TCF	T cell-specific transcription factor
TCR	T cell receptor
TGFb	Transforming growth factor beta
Th	T helper
TLR	toll-like receptor
TNF	tumor necrosis factor
T_{reg}	T regulatory cells
TUNEL	TdT-mediated dUTP-biotin nick end labeling
UC	ulcerative colitis
VEGF	vascular endothelial growth factor
VEGF	vascular endothelial growth factor
Wnt	mouse homolog of wingless

Common abbreviations may not be listed

Publications

Articles

1. ROS Production and NF-κB Activation Triggered by RAC1 Facilitate WNT-Driven Intestinal Stem Cell Proliferation and Colorectal Cancer Initiation.
K.B. Myant, P. Cammareri, E.J. McGhee, R.A. Ridgway, D.J. Huels, S. **Schwitalla**, G. Kalna, E.-L. Ogg, D. Athineos, P. Timpson, F.R. Greten, K.I. Anderson, O.J. Sansom
Cell Stem Cell 2013 Jun 6;12(6):761-73

2. Intestinal tumorigenesis initiated by dedifferentiation and acquisition of stem-cell-like properties.
S. Schwitalla, A.A. Fingerle, T. Nebelsiek, S.I. Göktuna, J. Heijmans, P. Cammareri, D.J. Huels, G. Moreaux, R.A. Rupec, M. Gerhard, R. Lang, J. Neumann, T. Kirchner, N. Barker, H. Clevers, O.J. Sansom, M.M. Taketo, G.R. van den Brink, M.C. Arkan and F.R. Greten
Cell 2013 Jan 17;152(1-2):25-38

3. Loss of p53 in enterocytes generates an inflammatory microenvironment enabling invasion and lymph node metastasis of carcinogen-induced colorectal tumors
S. Schwitalla, P. Ziegler, D. Horst, V. Becker, I. Kerle, Y. Begus-Nahrmann, A. Lechel, K.L. Rudolph, F.G. Bader, O. Prazeres da Costa, M.F. Neurath, A. Meining, T. Kirchner and F.R. Greten
Cancer Cell 2013 Jan 14;23(1):93-106

4. TNF-{alpha}-dependent loss of IKK{beta}-deficient myeloid progenitors triggers a cytokine loop culminating in granulocytosis
A.K. Mankan, O. Canli, **S. Schwitalla**, P. Ziegler, J. Tschopp, T. Korn and F.R. Greten
Proc Natl Acad Sci U S A 108(16):6567-6572 (2011)

5. Characterization of hybrid cells derived from spontaneous fusion events between breast epithelial cells exhibiting stem-like characteristics and breast cancer cells.
T. Dittmar, **S. Schwitalla**, J. Seidel, S. Haverkampf, G. Reith, S. Meyer-Staeckling, B. H Brandt, B. Niggemann, K.S. Zänker
Clinical & Experimental Metastasis. 28(1):75-90 (2010)

6. Recurrence cancer stem cells - Made by cell fusion?
T. Dittmar, C. Nagler, **S. Schwitalla**, G. Reith, B. Niggemann, K.S. Zänker
Medical Hypotheses 73(4):542-547 (2009)

7. gp130-Mediated Stat3 Activation in Enterocytes Regulates Cell Survival and Cell- Cycle Progression during Colitis-Associated Tumorigenesis.
J. Bollrath, T.J. Phesse, V.A. von Burstin, T. Putoczki, M. Bennecke, T. Bateman, T. Nebelsiek, T. Lundgren-May, O. Canli, **S. Schwitalla**, V. Matthews, R.M. Schmid, T. Kirchner, M.C. Arkan, M. Ernst and F.R. Greten
Cancer Cell 15(2):91-102 (2009)

8. Viscum Album extracts ISCADOR®P and ISCADOR®M counteract the growth factor induced effects in human follicular B-NHL cells and breast cancer cells.
F. Hugo, **S. Schwitalla**, B. Niggemann, K.S. Zänker, T. Dittmar
MEDICINA (Buenos Aires) 67: 90-96 (2007)

Book contribution

1. "one for all" or "all for one"?-The Necessity for Cancer Stem Cell Diversity in Metastasis formation and Cancer Relapse.
T. Dittmar, C. Nagler, **S. Schwitalla**, K. Krause, J. Seidel, G. Reith, B. Niggemann, K.S. Zänker
Stem Cell Biology in Health and Disease : pp 327-356 (2010)

2. Cancer Cell + Stem Cell= Cancer Stem Cell?
J. Seidel, E. Battistin, **S. Schwitalla**, T. Dittmar
New Cell Differentiation Research Topics: pp 117-152 (2007)
Articles

Danksagung

Herrn Prof. Dr. Florian Greten möchte ich dafür danken, dass er mir die Möglichkeit gegeben hat, in seiner Gruppe zu promovieren und dass ich diese spannenden und brisanten Projekte bearbeiten konnte. Ich habe im Verlauf dieser Arbeit unglaublich viel gelernt, prägende Erfahrungen gesammelt und konnte mich dadurch fachlich und auch persönlich weiterentwickeln. Florian Greten hat mich durch alle Phasen der Projekte hindurch hervorragend betreut, mich stets motiviert und unterstützt. Seine ständige Diskussionsbereitschaft, seine fachliche Kompetenz und Erfahrung haben essenziell zum Verlauf und zum Gelingen dieser Arbeit beigetragen. Danke für einfach alles, Florian!

Frau Prof. Dr. Angelika Schnieke danke ich ganz herzlich für die externe Betreuung meiner Promotion.

Ganz besonders möchte ich mich auch bedanken bei Kerstin Burmeister, Saskia Ettl, Julia Kaerlein und Kristin Retzlaff für ihre technische Unterstützung, die Labororganisation, Hilfe bei allen Tierstallangelegenheiten und besonders für einen außerordentlichen Job bei der Genotypisierung aller Mäuse. Ihr seid spitze!

Ebenso danke ich besonders Tiago deOliveira und auch Gülfem Öner für ihre großartige Leistung bei der Betreuung und dem Tailing der Mäuse in einem unserer Tierställe. You're fantastic, guys, thanks!

Ein herzlicher Dank geht natürlich auch an alle weiteren derzeitigen und auch ehemaligen Charaktere dieses Labors und an Dr. Canan Arkan und ihre Gruppe, die in jeder Situation ihre großartige Hilfsbereitschaft bewiesen und dem Labor mit ihrer freundschaftlichen Art eine wunderbare Atmosphäre verliehen haben: Özge Canli, Manon Schulz, Cigdem Atay, Franziska Romrig, Michaela Diamanti, Paul Ziegler, Charles Pallangyo, Julia Varga, Tiago deOliveira, Olga Goncharova, Hsin-Yu Fang, Jessica Heringer, Gülfem Öner, Abdel-Hamid Beji, Begüm Alankus, Dr. Julia Bollrath, Dr. Moritz Bennecke, Dr. Arun Mankan, Dr. Tim Nebelsiek, Dr. Serkan Göktuna und Dr. Jamil Khasawneh.
Danke, Teşekkürler, Asante, Ευχαριστω, Köszönöm, 多謝, شكرا, Obrigada, Merci, Спасибо!

Darüber hinaus will ich mich auch bei Prof. Dr. Owen Sansom und seinen Mitarbeitern Dr. Patrizia Cammareri und Dr. Kevin Myant für die

Kooperation und ihr Engagement sowie die Durchführung der *ex vivo* Versuche und Serientransplantationen bedanken, deren Daten in dieser Arbeit ebenfalls Verwendung gefunden haben.

Für die Bereitstellung des humanen Kollektivs möchte ich der Pathologie der TU München danken, sowie Frau Dr. Slotta-Huspenina und Ruth Wichnalek für die zügige Anfertigung der Paraffinschnitte.

Für die Durchführung der immunhistochemischen Analysen des humanen Kollektivs danke ich der Pathologie der LMU München und besonders Dr. David Horst für die fachmännische, pathologische Beurteilung der Fälle und die gute Zusammenarbeit.

Bei Dr. Valentin Becker und Irina Kerle will ich mich für die Ausführung der clsm-Analyse der Sunitinib-behandelten Tiere und für die quantitative, histolgische Auswertung der Tumor-Gefäßstrukturen bedanken.

Dr. Olivia Prazeres da Costa danke ich für die Durchführung und Analyse der Microarray Daten.

Allen Tierpflegern des ZPF danke ich für die gründliche Arbeit und ihre Fürsorglichkeit bei der Betreuung der Mäuse.

Außerdem möchte ich vor allem Berthold, Mieke, Marion, Caro, meinen Freunden und besonders meiner Oma und Luke dafür danken, dass sie immer für mich da sind.

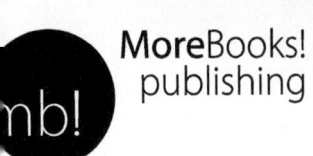
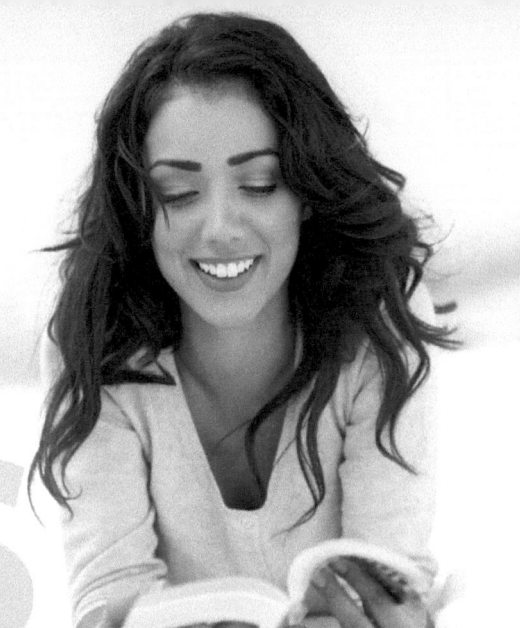

i want morebooks!

Buy your books fast and straightforward online - at one of world's fastest growing online book stores! Environmentally sound due to Print-on-Demand technologies.

Buy your books online at
www.get-morebooks.com

Kaufen Sie Ihre Bücher schnell und unkompliziert online – auf einer der am schnellsten wachsenden Buchhandelsplattformen weltweit! Dank Print-On-Demand umwelt- und ressourcenschonend produziert.

Bücher schneller online kaufen
www.morebooks.de

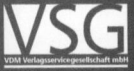

VDM Verlagsservicegesellschaft mbH
Heinrich-Böcking-Str. 6-8   Telefon: +49 681 3720 174   info@vdm-vsg.de
D - 66121 Saarbrücken   Telefax: +49 681 3720 1749 www.vdm-vsg.de

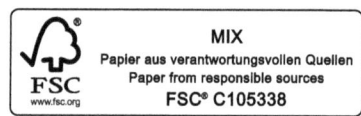

Printed by Books on Demand GmbH, Norderstedt / Germany